FUNCTIONAL APPLIANCES IN ORTHODONTIC TREATMENT

An atlas of clinical prescription and laboratory construction

FUNCTIONAL APPLIANCES IN ORTHODONTIC TREATMENT

An atlas of clinical prescription and laboratory construction

Harry S. Orton OBE

Introduction by
William R. Proffit

qb QUINTESSENCE PUBLISHING COMPANY
London, Chicago, Berlin, Tokyo, São Paulo & Hong Kong

First published 1990 by
Quintessence Publishing Company Ltd
London, UK
Second impression 1994
© 1990 Quintessence Publishing Co. Ltd
   and Harry S. Orton

British Library Cataloguing in Publication Data
Orton, Harry S.
 Functional appliances in orthodontic treatment.
 1. Man. Orthodontic appliances
 I. Title
 617.6430028

 ISBN 1-85097-012-2

Printed and bound in Great Britain by
Biddles Ltd, Guildford and King's Lynn.

To Shelagh

who steered this atlas to completion

This book as also been published in the following languages

German language
Funktionskierferorthopadische Gerate in der kieferorthopadischen
Behandlung
Quintessenz Verlags, Berlin.

Italian language
Gli Apparecchi Funzionali in Terapia Ortodontica
Indicazioni Cliniche e Tecniche di Costruzione.
Scienza e Tecnica Dentistica Edizioni Internazionali S.r.l. Milan.

Japanese language
現代ヨーロッパの
機能的矯正装置
その設計と処方
Quintessence Publishing Co Ltd
Tokyo, Japan.

INTRODUCTION TO THE SECOND IMPRESSION
by
Professor W.R. Proffit

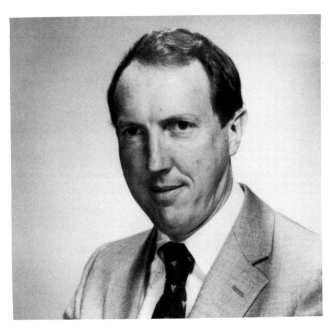

I am pleased that Harry Orton's *Functional Appliances in Orthodontic Treatment* has been well received and is now in its second impression. Also that editions have appeared in the German, Japanese and Italian languages.

My impression is that functional appliances are much less controversial now than they were when this book first appeared. The extreme advocates of functional appliances, who claimed improbable amounts of favorable growth in every case, by now have admitted that not all patients respond favorably. In fact, the best evidence at present suggests that 75-80% of children given a functional appliance show favorable differential growth – which means that 20-25% do not. Controlling undesirable tooth movement remains a key to successful treatment, especially when the growth response is minimal. The extreme detractors, who called the appliances not only useless but positively dangerous, have come to grudgingly admit that the appliances can facilitate mixed dentition treatment in selected cases. There still is room for a balanced view somewhere in between, which, along with its excellent illustrations of how the appliances are made and used, is what this book projects.

INTRODUCTION TO FIRST PRINTING

Harry Orton made the first of his several trips to Chapel Hill and the University of North Carolina in the late 1970s. We had heard that he was using a combination of fixed and functional appliances in an innovative way, and we were quite impressed with his continuing education course. It has been a real pleasure to visit him in Kingston since then and see the progress that he has made there, and to have Harry return to Chapel Hill to present new aspects of his work.

In many ways, the Kingston approach has combined the best of European functional appliance methods with the best of Anglo-American fixed appliance techniques. It is accepted now that one cannot provide comprehensive treatment with functional appliances alone. A second stage of fixed appliance treatment often (but not always) is needed, and that treatment must be available in a high-quality service. On the other hand, it also is clear now that a first stage of functional appliance treatment can greatly reduce the time and complexity of the later fixed appliance treatment, particularly in children with skeletal growth problems. For some patients, functional components can be combined with later fixed appliances to maintain maximum control.

The original proponents of functional appliances expected that they would stimulate growth of the mandible in mandibular-deficient Class II patients. It has been difficult to substantiate that claim. The changes from functional appliance treatment of Class II patients are due to a combination of four effects: (1) restraint of maxillary growth, similar to the effects of headgear; (2) acceleration of mandibular growth, so that the lower jaw grows faster for a time than otherwise would have been the case (even if it does not become much if any larger in the long run); (3) forward movement of lower teeth and retraction of upper teeth, similar to the effects of Class II elastics; and (4) rotation of the occlusal plane, with differential eruption of the lower molars and upper incisors. The first two effects produce differential growth of the jaws; the second two are antero-posterior and vertical tooth movement respectively.

To the extent possible, the orthodontist wants differential jaw growth from a functional appliance. Usually, tooth movement is not desired, particularly antero-posterior displacement of teeth. There are two keys to obtaining differential growth and minimizing dental effects. The first is using functional appliances only in patients who are growing. In the absence of growth, the only effect is tooth movement, but with good growth, differential growth usually will occur. For all practical purposes, this means that the appliances should be used in preadolescent children, not in older patients.

The second key is appliance design that controls the position of the teeth, for instance capping the lower incisors so that their forward movement is restricted. The fastest correction of a Class II malocclusion often is not the most effective functional appliance treatment, because quicker treatment usually includes a significant component of tooth movement. Maximizing skeletal change is slower and better.

Although it is possible to design functional appliances that incorporate major tooth-moving elements (screws and/or springs), often it is better to use separate appliances for tooth movement and growth guidance. For instance, in Class II Division 2 malocclusion, it is necessary to align the incisors before placing a functional appliance. This is done better either with a partial fixed appliance or a removable appliance designed for that purpose. Most Class II patients need some transverse expansion of the upper arch, and this too can be done advantageously for many patients with a separate expansion appliance before the functional appliance treatment begins. This atlas appropriately illustrates the design of removable appliances that would be used in preparation for functional treatment as well as the functional appliances themselves.

For some orthodontists, the controversy over whether functional appliances stimulate mandibular growth has obscured their genuine usefulness in mixed dentition treatment. It is not necessary for the appliances to make mandibles grow larger than they would have otherwise, in order to be quite valuable clinically. Nor is the undesirable tooth movement caused by some functional appliance designs an indictment of all functional appliances. Used correctly in the right patient, they can produce differential growth. Both patient selection and appliance design are important.

Harry Orton has contributed significantly to what I call the "components approach" to functional appliances, in which specific appliance components are selected to produce specific effects. Among other things, this atlas illustrates the effect of various components and shows how they can be combined in the treatment of common clinical situations. The components approach is particularly valuable when unusual patients are encountered, but it makes it easier to understand how an appliance would be modified under more common circumstances, as for instance when a mandibular deficient patient has anterior open bite as opposed to anterior deep bite.

I hope this atlas will prove valuable not only to students of orthodontics, but also to practitioners who have been reluctant to try modern functional appliance treatment – and I believe it will be.

WILLIAM R PROFFIT, DDS, PhD
Professor and Chairman
Department of Orthodontics
The University of North Carolina at Chapel Hill

CONTENTS

continued overleaf

CONTENTS (contd)

LIST OF PLATES

between pages   12 & 13

The plates show colour photographs, that are intended to compliment the drawings and text.
The clinical views are not intended to illustrate complete cases, but rather to show specific examples
of well made appliances and to give the reader a perspective of functional appliance dimension and
proportion. The *plates* will give the reader, who is unfamiliar with these appliances and this
diagnostic approach, a preview of the orthodontic philosophy encapsulated in this atlas.

Plate I   **Bite Taking and Impression Technique**

Plate II   **Expansion and Labial Segment Alignment Appliances (ELSAA's)**

Plate III   **ELSAA's (contd)**

Plate IV   **Activators**

Plate V   **Activators (contd)**

Plate VI   **'Intrusive' Functional Appliances**

Plate VII   **The Herbst Acrylic Splint**

Plate VIII   **The Function Regulators - Frankel Appliances (FR's)**

PREFACE TO SECOND IMPRESSION

The author has received many comments on the book and it has been most pleasing to see that it is seen as a valuable addition to orthodontic clinical knowledge. A number of readers have commented on the distilled and concentrated information on clinical management. This gives precise guidance on both the *strategy* of what is required in using functional appliances and also the *tactical detail* of "how to do it". A number of readers have seen it as the most practical book available on functional appliance thinking and usage.

Fixed appliances alone (which are excellent at *aligning* teeth) cannot handle the sagittal, vertical and lateral arch corrections that many occlusions need. A comprehensive orthodontic diagnostic treatment management programme requires a blending of functional, modern removable and fixed appliances.

A separate commentary on the value of the book is that publishing houses in Germany, Japan and Italy have independently decided that other language editions would benefit their populations. There is a growing international awareness of the value of functional appliances and the need to make them a part of the education and practice of all orthodontists.

PREFACE TO FIRST PRINTING

The use of orthodontic functional appliances at Kingston Hospital, Surrey, England, is and has been a process of continuing development since 1975. These appliances may be used as the sole means of treating an occlusal and facial problem but they are frequently blended into an edgewise fixed appliance system. Functional appliances are invariably used in the treatment of the most severe malocclusions. The principal criterion for the selection of functional appliances is whether or not the patient has any degree of profile handicap. Many previously treated cases have confirmed our early clinical impression that functional appliances handle the problems of facial misproportion better, and frequently more simply, than conventional orthodontic appliances. Correction of profile handicap sometimes occurs relatively rapidly (one year) with the standard construction of a well known appliance, or may occur slowly (2-3 years) and require frequent appliance remakes or changes in apparently inadequately complying patients. Great diagnostic, clinical and laboratory skill is needed for the prescription of an appliance that will be tolerated and work well.

The diagnostic approach to each case is based not only on the individual patient's requirements for occlusal and facial improvement, but also on the retrospective analysis of previous similar cases. This retrospective appreciation gives information on the human capacity for change and the capability of the various appliances to induce the required change. The appliance capability and patient's morphology have to be set within a social and institutional framework. Many of the systems are not only potent, but are also very simple. They are, however, totally dependent on the orthodontist's capacity for initial assessment, mid-course correction and particularly the ability to motivate the patients to co-operate.

Before the prescription of any functional appliance the orthodontist should undertake a component analysis. The clinician must know:

1. the components of the individual presenting occlusal and facial problem.
2. the components of expected growth for a similar patient.
3. the components of the many described functional appliances and what each of these functional appliance components will achieve either separately or in combination.

Having decided on an optimal prescription of appliance components for the patient's problem, the clinician then has to communicate his thinking to an informed technician who should try to understand the clinical consequences of his wire and acrylic placement. If possible one prescribes standard appliances, but the appliance must fit the problem not the other way round. After the functional component analysis, do not hesitate, in discussion with the technician, to personalise the functional appliance to make it fully appropriate to the patient's clinical problem.

However apt the design and construction of an appliance, **patient tolerance is all**. If the patient cannot be motivated to wear the appliance for the greater part of the day and night, it will not work. It is better to underprescribe or underactivate and have the appliance worn, than prescribe, what is for the particular patient, an ideal but poorly tolerated appliance.

I should like to acknowledge our indebtedness to many previous orthodontists whose ideas have been the foundation for this development. In particular I should like to single out Dr. Rolf Fränkel for his unique and special contribution. I would hope that he would not feel aggravated by the small changes we have made to his appliances. The range of activators is descended from Andreson via Harvold and Mew. The Range of expansion and labial segment alignment appliances (ELSAA'S) has developed from the Mew 1 appliance. This Atlas does not set out to be a comprehensive overview of all the functional appliances that have ever been described. Rather, it is a compendium of functional appliances that have been shown to work in the hands of supervised trainee orthodontists. **These appliance systems will enable any skilled orthodontist to treat any moderate to severe Class II malocclusion that presents, provided that the face is growing and the patient can be motivated to cooperate.**

A functional component analysis (ie patient need and appliance capability) is an essential preliminary to the design of a functional appliance, but **it must be followed by good laboratory support**. I would like to acknowledge my indebtedness to our two senior chief technicians, Bill Johnston and Bill Keel, who have coped with my 'mid-course corrections' for many years.

The Princess Dental Wing at Kingston Hospital, Kingston-upon-Thames, Surrey, UK

HARRY S. ORTON, OBE

Consultant Orthodontist to:
Kingston Hospital, Surrey; The Eastman Dental Hospital; St Thomas's Hospital; The British Army; and in Private Practice in Surbiton, Surrey

WHEN TO PRESCRIBE A FUNCTIONAL APPLIANCE

Each of the 3 main treatment modalities of orthodontics has, in average clinical use, the strengths and weaknesses that are outlined below. When presented with an individual patient problem, the clinician should undertake a 'component analysis' of the presenting morphology, the capacity for, and direction of probable growth, and the treatment required to correct the patient's occluso-facial problem. The complete orthodontist should be able to deploy, singly or in combination, the fixed, modern removable, or functional appliances needed to solve the patient's problem. The table below gives broad guidance on the strengths and weaknesses of our three major treatment systems in the solution of occluso-facial problems.

	Edgewise Appliance	Modern Removables	Functional Appliances
Individual Tooth Positioning	E	P	P
Torquing	G-A	P	P
Arch formation	G-A	A-P	A
Intercuspation	A	A-P	A
Lateral Expansion	A-P	E	G-A
En Masse Movement	A-P	E+Headgear	G+Headgear
Sagittal Arch Correction	A-P	G+Headgear	E-G
Vertical Maxillary Control	A-P	E-G+Headgear	E-G (correct system)
Avoidance of Gingival & Root Morbidity	A-P	G-A	E

E = excellent   G = good   A = average   P = poor

The atlas as a whole gives detailed guidance on the appropriateness and design of a particular functional appliance for the solution of a specific area of clinical presentation.

THE LAYOUT OF EACH CHAPTER

Each of the five main chapters will have some pages of introductory text. The purpose of this text is to give an overview of the place of the appliance system within the spectrum of orthodontic treatment. The detail of each appliance within the five systems is shown on the right hand page in diagrammatic form. Above each set of diagrams is set out the 'Functional Component Objectives' sought for that particular appliance. On the left hand page the **clinician** will find clinical guidance on the prescription of that particular appliance for the appropriate clinical category of patient, as well as the design, the clinical records needed, and the visit by visit treatment expectations and requirements. On the same page, the **technician** will find guidance on the construction of that appliance. Both clinician and technician should, with advantage, study the other's text. Where the amount of combined clinical and technical text is too much for one page, then the technical guidance for that particular appliance is continued on the following page, but with a repeat of the appropriate diagram page. On all diagrams wire sizes are shown in millimetres, with the appropriate USA gauge size equivalent shown at the bottom of each appliance design card. A more comprehensive wire size conversion chart is printed at the end of chapter six.

THE FUNCTIONAL APPLIANCE DESIGN CARD

Clinical guidance on completion of the card

- A basic decision on the appropriateness of a functional appliance to the patient's facial and occlusal problem should have been made at the diagnostic and parental discussion visit. During this visit full records should be presented to the parents. It also helps to establish confidence by showing the records of similar successfully treated functional appliance cases.

- At this diagnostic visit a preliminary choice of functional appliance system should be made, since this will affect the time allowed and the materials prepared for the first treatment visit.

- At the first treatment visit the order of work should be:
  1. **To confirm that the type of functional appliance previously chosen** is the most appropriate appliance for the malocclusion, and in particular **to study the detail of any tooth misplacement** which may indicate minor variations in wire and acrylic positioning.
  2. **To draw and write an accurate description** of the functional appliance that the clinician has chosen on a functional appliance design card. This is crucial for effective communication with and motivation of the technician. It also serves to concentrate the mind of the clinician. A specimen of the type of card used in the Princess Dental Wing of Kingston Hospital is printed opposite.
  3. **To obtain an accurate bite.** This is the most crucial step in the construction of a functional appliance and will vary from one type of appliance to another, and to a smaller extent from patient to patient. The detail of these variations in bite taking will be discussed for each separate appliance system.
  4. **Lastly, to take the working impressions.** Again impression techniques may vary from one system to another. These variations will also be discussed for each separate appliance system.

- This order of work is frequently reversed by many clinicians and may result in failing to obtain an accurate bite on a patient who is already unsettled by the impression taking. It can also result in rushing the most important, quiet, contemplative, functional component analysis, that should precede the design of an appliance that is appropriate for the individual patient's facial and occlusal problem.

Technical guidance on receipt of the card

- It is in the longterm interests of the technician that the clinician's functional appliance treatment plans should succeed.

- This can only occur if the patient is presented with the correctly designed appliance, that is made to the correct bite and is of a tolerable size and quality of finish for that patient.

- This requires the technician not only to be technically expert, but **to understand how the appliance works** and **to be able to assess the accuracy of the clinical records.**

- Unfortunately many clinicians do not complete appliance cards at all well, nor may they have fully thought through the design.

- On-going education, rapport and communication between clinician & technician and technician & clinician, is vital to obtaining the best from functional appliances.

Functional Component Objectives	Practice/Clinic/Hospital	
	Patient's Name & Number	
	Impression Date	**Date for Finish**
	Clinician	**Technician**

FUNCTIONAL APPLIANCE DESIGN CARD FOR A .....

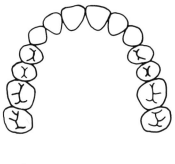

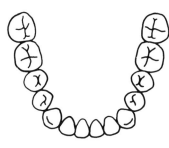

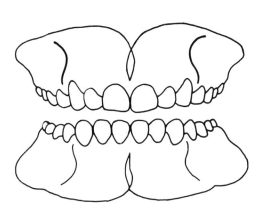

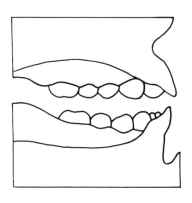

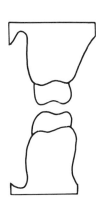

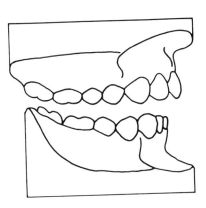

Wire specifications;

INTRODUCTION TO THE COLOUR PLATES

Before the second world war each country and even continent tended to have its own separate style of orthodontics. The Europeans developed the original functional appliance systems, the Americans (USA) developed the fixed appliance systems particularly the edgewise appliance, the British initially concentrated on the removable appliance with active spring components, the labio-lingual systems were common to all. Australasia saw the separate development of the Begg fixed appliance system.

The 60s, 70s and 80s, with their explosion of information exchange, educational opportunity, travel facilities, and in particular the larger number of innovative suppliers of orthodontic materials, saw an increasingly rapid cross-fertilisation of international orthodontic practice. There is still, however, a tendency for some practitioners to continue to search for, and to try to adopt the illusory single technique which will answer most, or even all of their orthodontic problems. There is, of course, no such orthodontic technique panacea and the diversity of patient need and our ability to think and respond flexibly is the strength of the profession. A study of the recent history of orthodontics reveals an astonishing and ever-shortening 'half-life of knowledge in orthodontics' and with it the consequent requirement for each practitioner and technician to remain in an evolving senior student mode during the whole of their practicing lives.

It is the author's belief that the next decade of advance in **the treatment of serious Class II malocclusion** will be with **the skillful and INTEGRATED use of functional and modern removable appliances with the edgewise appliance** during the period of facial growth. This approach requires the practitioner to be above all **a wise planner of treatment** and also to know the strengths and weaknesses of the separate components that are being integrated. The overall orthodontic treatment aim should be **to achieve the most for doing the least.** Being over-busy and over-complex for over-long, frequently results in iatrogenic damage or burnt-out patients.

A number of the following patient-proven and recommended appliance systems may be unfamiliar to some readers. The colour photographs will firstly allow an appliance to be related to its name. It will secondly give an idea of the appliance's form and function in the mouth. The legends are intended to illustrate a clinical scenario which may be personally familiar to the reader. The reader can then think how that clinical problem might be solved with the clinician's current approach and compare the alternative solution that is suggested in the legend. The legends are cross referenced to the appropriate Design Card or text so that the reader can be selectively led into the atlas before studying the text in its entirety. These colour plates become effectively a book within a book.

Do study the detail of the appliances since it is often critical as to how well the treatments work.

- *Plate I.* - On Bites and Impression Technique stresses the need to seek only a small activation of the bite for the first functional appliance in order to obtain maximised patient tolerance. Functional appliances should be progressively advanced.

- *Plate II.* - On Expansion and Labial Segment Alignment Appliances (ELSAA'S) shows the more commonly used designs and their alignment capability.

- *Plate III.* - ELSAA'S (continued) shows appliances with and without anterior alignment wires for treating Class II Division 2 occlusions and mid-arch extraction cases.

- *Plate IV.* - Shows the commonly used Activators of the Medium Opening Activator-Palatal and the Medium Opening Activator-Labial types.

- *Plate V.* - Activators (continued) shows variants of the Medium Opening Activators used in combination with fixed appliances.

- *Plate VI.* - Shows Intrusive Functional Appliances aimed at posterior maxillary intrusion, whole arch maxillary intrusion and maxillary intrusion combined with two techniques for mandibular advancement.

- *Plate VII.* - Shows the Herbst Acrylic Splint laterally, upper and lower splints occlusally, and the splints functioning in the mouth.

- *Plate VIII.* - Shows the Function Regulators (Frankel Appliances) as they are used in the Princess Dental Wing at Kingston Hospital, Surrey, England.

BITE - TAKING AND IMPRESSION TECHNIQUE

See all Chapters, Design Cards 1-3, 8A-11, 13-18

N.B. Firstly DESIGN the appliance, secondly take the BITE, thirdly take the IMPRESSIONS (see page 10).

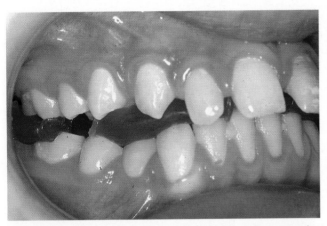

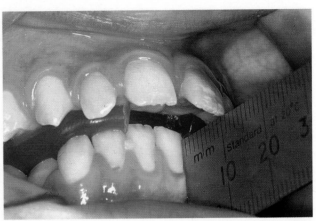

Ia. Patient C.B, timid boy aged 9.10 years, 15mm overjet, overbite complete, ‖ recently badly concussed, vital but greying. Overjet reduction needed to reduce accident risk, with minimal pressure on ‖. A **Buccal window cut** in a horseshoe of Tenatex wax **visualises the vertical opening. Articulated, it is always 1mm more than seen in the mouth.** ie 2-2.5mm bite opening is plenty for the first functional.

Ib. Patient C.B, anxious boy who will need to be cosseted along. A small capped Frankel prescribed, 4mm is enough for a **tolerable initial advance of the bite** (see ruler). The **anterior window allows the centre-lines to be checked**. The Frankel can easily be advanced 1.5 to 2mm at 4 months and again at 8 months prior to a second larger Frankel on, by then, an experienced Frankel patient (*Plate VIIIe*).

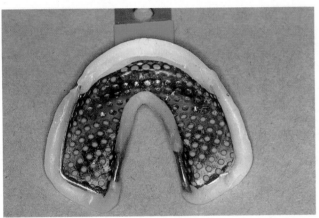

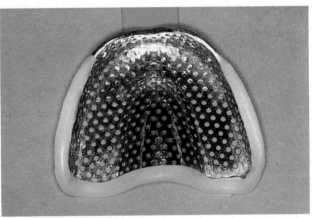

Ic. AFTER taking the bite, THEN take the impressions. **Preparation of the LOWER tray** - Choose a tray tending to small rather than large. Seek vertical distention of the vestibule. Do not bottom out on the lingual of the lower labial segment, use a lingual ring of firm beading wax. Two labial wax strips on the inside of tray (not needed for activators) are shown for a Class II Frankel, (see page 16).

Id. **Preparation of the UPPER tray** - It should be a more generous fit than the lower particularly antero-posteriorly with procumbent upper incisors. The author prefers Coe perforated trays. Waxing shown for a Class II Frankel (no buccal waxing for activators). Use a dust free alginate with good flow AND body. Seat trays well vertically with gentle outward & downward stretching of the lips and cheeks.

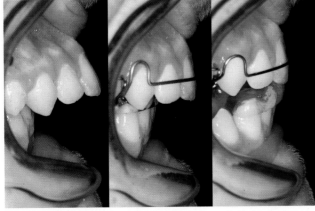

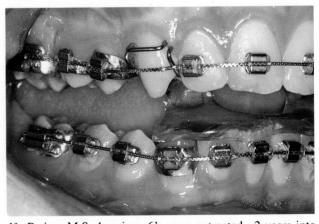

Ie. Overjet at the start of active treatment   Overjet in the FIRST activator   Overjet in the SECOND activator

Patient M.S, male aged 12.6 years, starting overjet 15mm showing **progressive bite advance** for maximised functional appliance tolerance.

If. Patient M.S, 4 carious 6's were extracted. 2 years into treatment (1yr functional, 1yr functional+fixed), overjet is now 2mm. **The sagittal arch correction is maintained** with a modified Medium Opening Activator-Labial (see page 45) during the first year of fixed therapy. For this THIRD activator **the bite is edge to edge**. The functional appliance is discarded for the final fixed appliance detailing.

Plate I

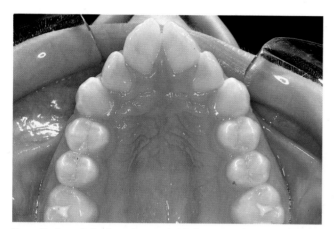

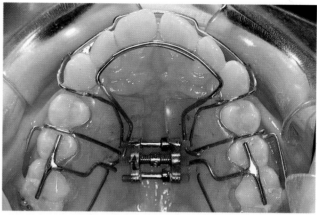

IIa. Patient J.A, female aged 10.5 years, Class II Div 1, overjet 9mm, overbite complete. **Here, at diagnosis**, she is seen to need 5mm expansion of 6|6, 3mm expansion of 3|3, alignment and derotation of 21|12. An ELSAA is prescribed to achieve this before going on to a Medium Opening Activator - Palatal (MOA-Palatal), see Design Card 8A (DC 8A), page 37.

IIb. Patient J.A, after 4 months of treatment wearing **the most commonly used ELSAA**, (see DC 4 i, page 25). The labial insets on 2|2 were produced with a triple beak plier by the clinician. The palatal incisal alignment wires are stiff, gently activated 'nudgers'.

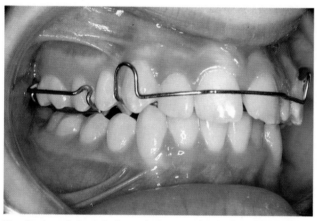

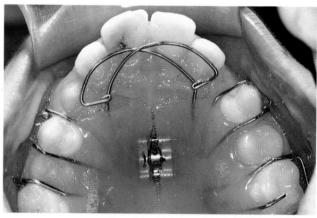

IIc. Patient J.A, right lateral view, at 4 months of treatment, showing **the buccal overjet and approximate incisor alignment** which will accomodate the forward positition of the mandible in the activator phase. Note the double crib on 65| and highish labial bow position. The midline screw is now fused, to maintain expansion when the MOA-Palatal activator is out of the mouth (see page 34).

IId. Patient M.R, male aged 11 years, overjet 7mm, overbite complete, 1|1 are already damaged. He needs lateral buccal expansion and minor labial movement of 2|2 prior to a MOA-Palatal. **The more flexible palatal incisal alignment wires** are similar to DC 4 iv, page 25.

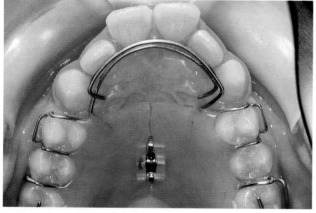

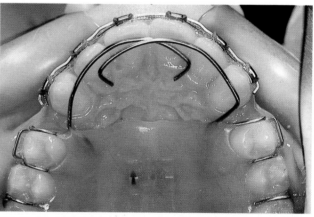

IIe. Patient O.W, male aged 10.5 years, overjet 13mm, overbite complete to palate. He requires labial consolidation of 2|2 on 1|1 position, but also mesio-distal consolidation of 321|123. The palatal wires embody features of the ELSAA in DC 4 iii & iv, page 25.

IIf. Patient O.W, after 3 months of **ELSAA treatment plus anterior brackets** (3|3 bonded at 3 weeks). Note the spare wire take-up. The screw is fused prior to a MOA-Labial with brackets, see *Plate Va & b* and page 49.

Plate II

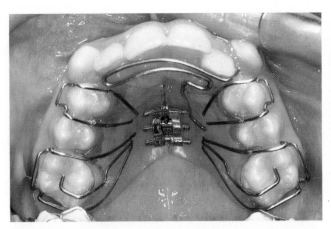

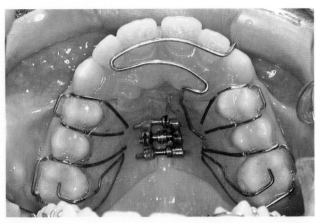

IIIa. Patient J.A, female aged 13.8 years, 6 months past menarchy. Class II Div 2, moderately increased overbite, 3/12 immediate history of serious TMJ dysfunction, 4x7s extracted. ELSAA prescribed (see DC 5 ii, page 27) to expand buccally, align the labial segment by proclination and **create an overjet to facilitate the use of a MOA-Palatal,** (see DC 8A, page 37).

IIIb. Patient J.A, 4 months into treatment showing the **design of ELSAA commonly used for treating Class II Div 2 malocclusion.** TMJ pain gone, 6|6 expanded 5mm, 3|3 accommodated in the arch, some distal movement of 6|6, 21|12 aligned, 1|1 axially corrected, 8mm of overjet created, prior to using the MOA-Palatal.

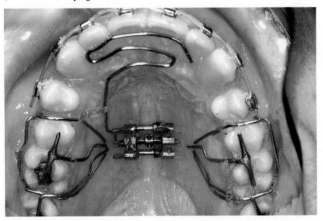

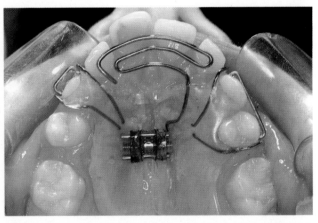

IIIc. Patient C.P, physically immature male aged 16.5 years, with a Class II intermediate incisal relationship, increased overbite and a mildly crowded upper labial segment. An **ELSAA + labial brackets prescribed** (see DC 5 ii, page 27) to create an aligned consolidated overjet prior to using a MOA-Palatal + anterior brackets (see DC 9 ii, page 43).

IIId. Patient A.L, female, aged 12.1 years, Class II Div 1, 8mm overjet with profile handicap, **but needing mid-arch relief of crowding,** 4x5s were extracted. An ELSAA (see DC 7 ii, page 31) used to round instanding 2|12 forward, retract 3|34 reciprocally, reduce 5|5 spaces, expand 3|34 but not 4| prior to the use of a MOA-Labial, (see DC 10 ii, page 45).

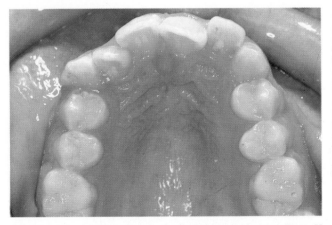

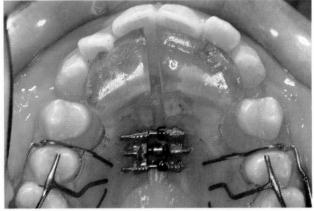

IIIe. Patient A.P, big female aged 12 years, marked Class II Div 2 profile and incisal relationship, mid-arch extractions contra-indicated but severe U/L labial segment crowding present, 4x7s were extracted. **At the start of treatment,** upper (and lower) incisal alignment is needed, with some distal movement and expansion of the Class II upper buccal segments.

IIIf. Patient A.P, after 9 months of treatment using two appliances in which **the acrylic anterior bite-plate and screw are the active intra-oral components** (see DC 6 ii, page 29) but with headgear applied to the bridges of the 6|6 cribs. Together, these have produced a mild Class III buccal occlusion, a reduced overbite, some labial tipping of 1|1 and adequate space for fixed appliance occlusal detailing.

Plate III

ACTIVATORS

See CHAPTER THREE, Design Cards 8A & 10, pages 37 &45

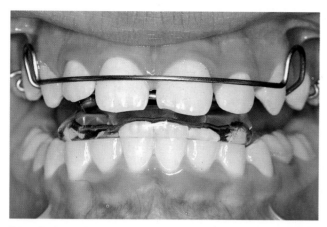

IVa. Patient J.L, robust boy aged 10.3 years, 11mm overjet, overbite complete to palate, facially retrognathic. He was treated non-extraction, initially with an ELSAA. The photograph shows the front of his **MEDIUM OPENING ACTIVATOR PALATAL** (see DC 8A, page 37), the labial bow and palatal wire are positioned well, **the lower labial segment capping should ideally be 1mm deeper.**

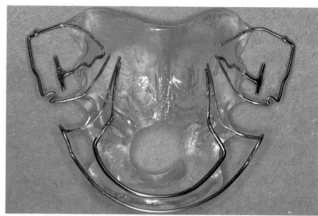

IVb. Patient J.L's MOA-Palatal viewed from the palatal surface. The double cribs are neatly made with good sized, well angulated arrowheads and butterfly occlusal rests. The wire ends are neatly placed in the acrylic. The labial wire is ideal in form, the palatal wire is a trifle too shaped. **The anterior breathing hole should be larger than this if structurally possible.**

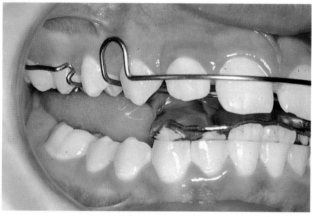

IVc. Patient J.L's MOA-Palatal in the mouth, showing good positioning of 5| arrowhead AT the gingival margin. The labial wire is AT the tips of the interdental papillae and the palatal wire is TOWARDS the incisal tips. The bite is 5-6mm forwards, **but is 1-2mm too open for reliable tolerance in many patients,** (see *Plate 1a*).

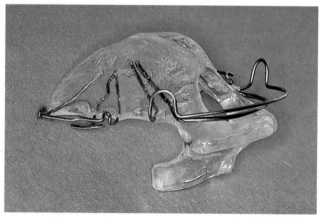

IVd. Patient J.L's MOA-Palatal in side view showing the vertical relationship of the occlusal rest to the double crib and the palatal wire to the labial bow. **There is no vertical or lingual constraint of the lower buccal segment teeth.** The corners of the lingual mandibular guidance flanges are too square and need rounding, (see below *Plate IVf*).

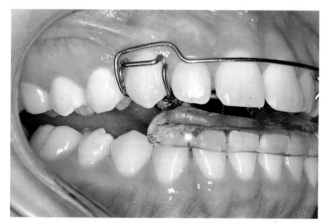

IVe. Patient V.B, pubertal female aged 12.2 years, Class II Div 2, a full crown of overbite, mild crowding, 4x7s were extracted. An ELSAA + brackets 3+3 , converted her to a Class II Div 1 but induced upper buccal segment spacing. 3|3 brackets were removed and (see DC 10, page 45) a **MEDIUM OPENING ACTIVATOR-LABIAL** cribbed on 3|3 was fitted. 21|12 brackets were removed later.

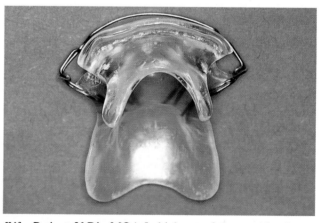

IVf. Patient V.B's MOA-Labial out of the mouth, shown from a mandibular aspect. The outline of the spoon palate can be seen together with an inside view of the lower labial segment capping. This is smoothly polished on the mucosal surface but with precise contact on the lower incisor tips. The lingual mandibular guidance flanges are nicely rounded. If a flange fractures later, just smooth it off.

Plate IV

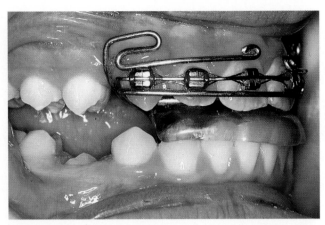

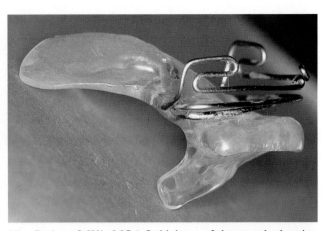

Va. Patient O.W. (see *Plate IIe & f* for his history and ELSAA usage) has a 13mm overjet with profile handicap and aligned 3＋3 with spacing between 4|4 and 3|3. A **MEDIUM OPENING ACTIVATOR - LABIAL with anterior brackets** (see DC 11, page 49) is prescribed. The 3＋3 bow, incisal to the brackets, retracts the labial segment to the buccal segments.

Vb. Patient O.W's MOA-Labial out of the mouth showing the spoon palate, the lower labial capping, the mandibular guidance flanges, thr labial bow (without 'U' loops) and the flexible retention clips lying gingival to the brackets. The retention arms are overlong and need only extend to the mesial of 2|2.

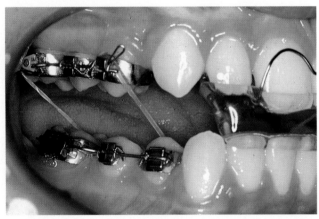

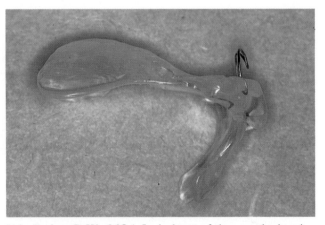

Vc. Patient R.K, a cooperative boy aged 11.10 years, 14mm overjet, complete overbite, treated with an ELSAA and two medium opening activators to an overjet of 3.5mm but the buccal segment eruption was slow. A **MEDIUM OPENING ACTIVATOR-INCISAL** maintains the sagittal correction but is **opened vertically** for buccal extrusion and crossbite guidance with vertical elastics.

Vd. Patient R.K's MOA-Incisal out of the mouth showing the spoon palate, the upper and lower incisor capping, the lingual mandibular guidance flanges, and the incisal wire (see page 68) for retention and to minimise 1|1 tipping. This appliance **must be heat-cured** and is only appropriate for the experienced activator wearer. Appliance strength does not permit an anterior breathing hole.

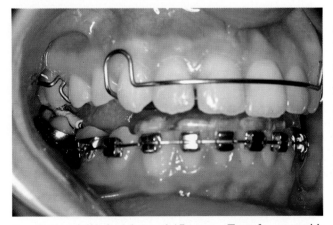

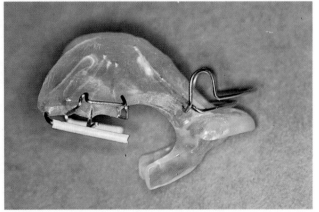

Ve. Patient S.W, female aged 17 years. Transfer case with 6|6 previously extracted. 7|7 badly tipped, substantial TMJ pain dysfunction, mildly crowded Class II incisal relationship. 7|7 were extracted and ELSAA therapy (4 months) + lower fixed started, prior to a **MOA-Palatal with posterior occlusal stops** to control extrusion of 7|7. This treatment succeeded in spite of the patient's age.

Vf. Patient S.W's MOA-Palatal, showing the profile of the appliance with acrylic trimmed around 54|45 to permit their unimpeded vertical development. 6|6 and 7|7 are controlled vertically, 6|6 by the occlusal rest and crib, and 7|7 by the 1mm occlusal bar, covered with heat-shrunk plastic. 7|7 uprighted easily, without extrusion, using a series of rectangular Nickel Titanium levelling arches.

Plate V

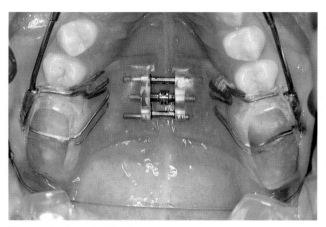

VIa. Patient D.T, female aged 15.1 years, overlate presentation for treatment, 10mm overjet, anterior open bite extending forwards from the first molars, intermittent thumbsucking, moderate lower anterior face height. Intrusion and expansion of 76|67 and intrusion of 76|67, using a **BUCCAL INTRUSION SPLINT (BIS)** + intrusive headgear (see DC 14, page 63).

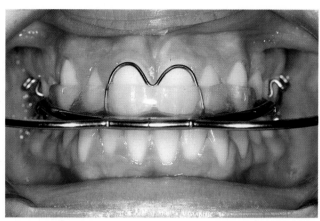

VIb. Patient C.C, female aged 13.1 years, moderate skeletal II base, mild crowding, 7mm overjet, gummy bimaxillary protrusion. Loss of lower premolars and over-uprighting of lower incisors would worsen the facial appearance, 8s well positioned, so 4x7s were extracted. An ELSAA was used prior to this standard **MAXILLARY INTRUSION SPLINT (MIS)** (see DC 15, page 67).

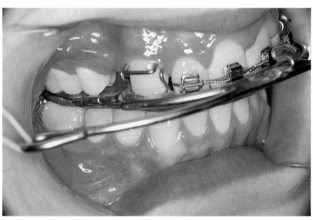

VIc. Patient J.C, early pubertal female aged 11.10 years, very gummy Class II Div 1, acute naso-labial angle, overjet 11.5mm, increased overbite, very spaced 21|12. Previous unwanted loss of 4|4. Consolidation forwards of 321|123 using an ELSAA + anterior brackets, left 10 mm of space in 4|4 region. **Tunnel plastering**, of 7654|4567, **within a MIS**, allowed 4|4 space closure (see pages 66 & 68).

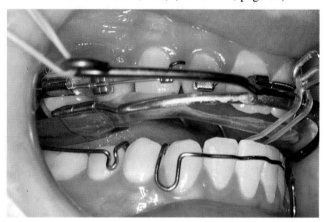

VId. Patient J.C, 4|4 space was closed in 1 year. 65|56 are now bonded, and forward mandibular displacement has been induced by using **the Concorde hook on the Kloehn whisker** (see page 70) to a **Clark type lower traction plate** (see page 71).

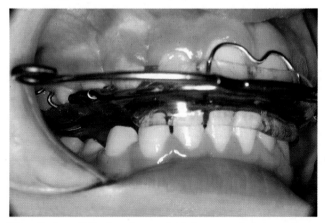

VIe. Patient C.R, female aged 10.3 years, slightly gummy Class II Div 1, overjet 10.5mm, overbite complete to palate, facially retrognathic. An ELSAA was used prior to an **INTRUSIVE ACTIVATOR** (see page 75). Note the 'flying headgear tube' (see page 68), short whisker and occlusal plastering on 54|. The first bite is only 3-4mm forward to maximise patient tolerance.

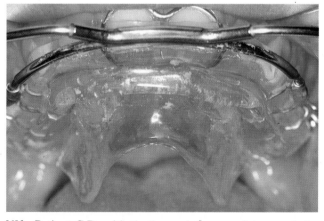

VIf. Patient C.R, with the lower jaw opened to reveal the thin rounded smooth lingual flanges of the intrusive activator. The occlusal shelf is smooth and in contact with the tips of the cusps of the lower buccal segment teeth only, (the fissures are plastered out on the working model).

Plate VI

THE HERBST ACRYLIC SPLINT

See CHAPTER FIVE Design Card 18, pages 87-91

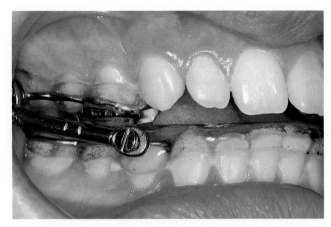

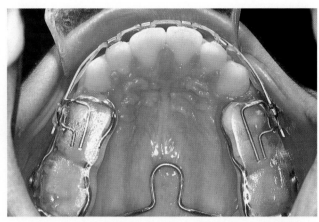

VIIa. Patient J.M, mature young male, aged 13.9 years, Class II Div 1, 11mm overjet, failed activator case (see page 78). The start of Herbst treatment shows a **standard HERBSTACRYLICSPLINT** (page 87). Note the depth of the lower labial capping and the slightly under-extended buccal capping which **should be** just 1mm clear of the buccal gingival margins.

VIIb. Patient S.A, early pubertal female aged 12.8 years, 14mm overjet, very spaced upper incisors. Failed MIS + headgear, failed capped Frankel. Then treated to an overjet of 3mm with this **upper bonded Herbst acrylic splint** showing closure of the upper labial segment spacing using anterior brackets, AFTER the lower splint was loosened (page 83, Retention Methodology).

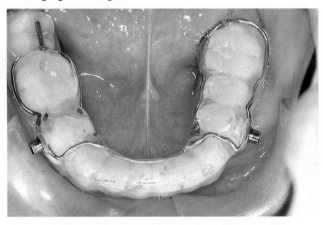

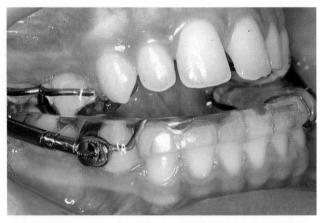

VIIc. Patient C.S, female aged 13.4 years, at boarding school, 10mm overjet, high FMPA, very incomplete overbite, right second premolars congenitally absent. Treatment with a BIS plus headgear failed. The occlusal view of a **lower Herbst acrylic splint** shows the general splint form, lower axles and occlusal stop on $\overline{7I}$.

VIId. Patient C.S, right lateral view of upper and lower acrylic splints. Class III incisal relationship achieved after 5 months of Herbst treatment. **Progressive advance of the piston with the use of buccal washers** can be seen (page 82, Clinical Management). The AOB closed with removal of the buccal overlays. U/L fixed appliances + Class II traction then used to tidy up the occlusion.

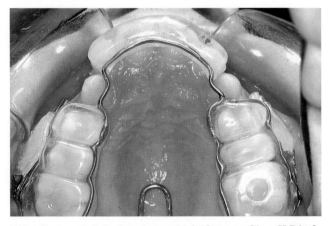

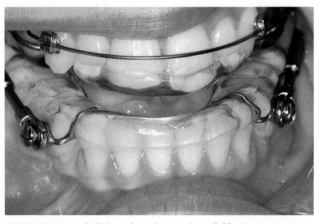

VIIe. Patient C.C-L, female aged 16.10 years, Class II Div 2, crowded upper labial segment, moderate palatal impaction of unerupted $3I$ and a bilabially concave profile. An ELSAA proclined $\underline{21I12}$ prior to a MOA-Pal which was not worn well and then lost. $3I$ spontaneously erupted. This occlusal view of the upper splint with incisal capping has a **palatal bypass wire** around $3I3$ (see page 79).

VIIf. Patient C.C-L, after 6 months of Herbst treatment, is **here protruding the mandible**, to show 6-7mm of piston which could **now accept a second buccal washer**. $3I3$ roots are being torqued buccally with a rounded-edge rectangular wire.

Plate VII

THE FUNCTION REGULATORS - FRANKEL APPLIANCES (FR's)

See CHAPTER ONE, Design Cards 1-3, pages 17-21

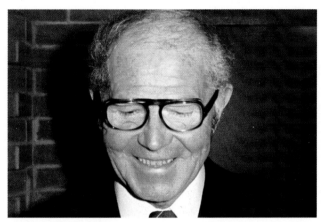

VIIIa. **Prof em Dr Rolf Fränkel** was born in Leipzig on March 29, 1908. He has been an outstanding contributor to functional appliance thought and is the creator of the Function Regulator (Frankel) System of appliances. This photograph was taken whilst he was lecturing in Manchester, England in 1975.

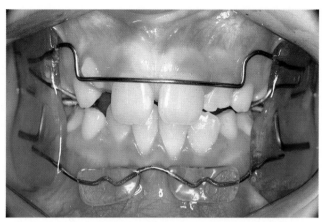

VIIIb. Patient J.F, female aged 8.11 years, Class II Div 1, early mixed dentition, overjet of 11mm and mild lower incisor crowding. She was treated with this **FRANKEL APPLIANCE for Class II Div 1 occlusions with normal or reduced overbites** (page 17). Note the buccal shield and pelote form and position, together with the shape and position of the wires.

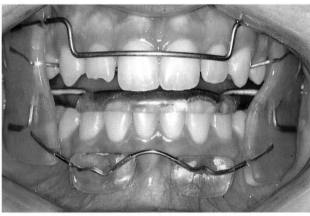

VIIIc. Patient E.S, male aged 11.6 years, Class II Div 2, full crown of incisor overbite, lowish FMPA. 4x7s were extracted, an ELSAA used to convert to a Class II Div 1 incisor relationship prior to a **FRANKEL APPLIANCE with LOWER INCISAL CAPPING** (page 18). Note the capping of the lower labial segment, the shape and position of wires, buccal shields and lower labial pelotes.

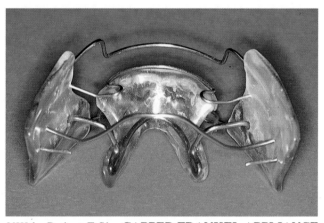

VIIId. Patient E.S's, **CAPPED FRANKEL APPLIANCE** photographed from behind showing the lower labial segment capping, the lingual hanger and lingual guidance flanges, the rounded edges and smooth inner sweep of the buccal shields, the occlusal rests on 6|6, and the transpalatal, anterior-palatal, and labial wires (page 19).

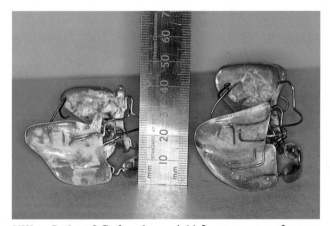

VIIIe. Patient J.C, female aged 11.2 years, a transfer case with 4x4s already extracted, all spaces closed, 10mm of residual overjet, a smallish rima oris, and a retrognathic profile. She was treated successfully with these two Frankels, in 1976/77. Though old fashioned in design, they illustrate a **small initial appliance for tolerance**, followed by a larger, more demanding FR, 11 months later.

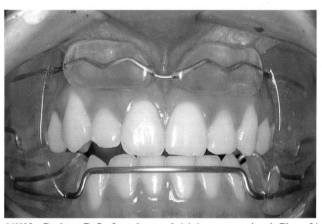

VIIIf. Patient D.S, female aged 14.1 years, mixed Class I/ Class III, underlying Skeletal III base. Treated with upper lateral+sagittal expansion, and headgear to a lower removable appliance. Relapse tendency controlled with a **FRANKEL APPLIANCE for Class III occlusions with 'Kingston' modified buccal shields** (see page 21). **This appliance is best used in the early mixed dentition.**

Plate VIII

CHAPTER ONE

THE FUNCTION REGULATORS - FRANKEL APPLIANCES (FR's) DESIGN CARDS 1-3

The comprehensive function regulator system designed by Rolf Fränkel has in over a decade been refined down to three appliances at Kingston Hospital.

PRESCRIPTION FOR THE CLASS II FRANKEL APPLIANCE

The Class II Frankel (Design Card 1) is prescribed for average Frankfort-Mandibular Planes Angle (FMPA), normal to reduced overbite, mild to moderate skeletal discrepancy, relatively aligned arches in Class II Division 1 occlusions with profile retrognathia.

The capped Class II Frankel (Design Card 2) is prescribed for average to low FMPA, increased or deep and complete overbites, mild to moderate skeletal discrepancy, relatively aligned arches in Class II Division 1 occlusions with profile retrognathia.

Neither of these appliances is particularly appropriate for the very severe (12-14 mm+) overjet and the potentially timorous patient, who is more easily managed in the initial stages of treatment with a medium opening activator. Neither appliance is appropriate for the higher Frankfurt Mandibular Plane Angle (FMPA) patient. Both appliances work well through the whole of the mixed dentition period and into the early permanent dentition. Since the appliances are largely tissue borne they produce little interference with the natural exfoliation of the primary dentition and are frequently readily tolerated by the young patient. The more mature the full permanent dentition becomes, the less well the appliances (1 and 2) work. The FR's allow some maxillary arch expansion (approximately 3.5mm on 6|6 and 2mm on 3|3) and rounding out to take place within the buccal shields and the labial wires. There is therefore no need in most cases for **preliminary** maxillary arch alignment and expansion using a removable expansion and labial segment alignment appliance (ELSAA). If, however, there is a buccal segment crossbite and/or there are very instanding upper lateral incisors, **these should be corrected first.** If an ELSAA is used as the initial appliance, then the ELSAA must then be worn when the FR is out of the mouth for the first four months of Frankel therapy. For long-term occlusal stability it is better to avoid lower arch expansion. For this reason the inner lower portion of the buccal shield has a relief which allows free eruption of the lower buccal segments but little space for lower buccal expansion. However, the longer FR therapy continues ie 1 year+, the more lower arch expansion takes place.

EFFECT ON THE FACIAL SKELETON

The superimposed tracings (De Coster's line and the fine bony detail of anterior cranial base) of many cases, during an average period of treatment, has shown:

- Sagittal maxillary arrest.

- No significant change in the Y-axis.

- A change in the ratio of descent of the maxilla : mandible from 1:1 to 1:2.

- This vertical downward acceleration of the mandible, with no opening of the Y-axis and maxillary sagittal arrest, gives a consistent reduction in the Class II apical base discrepancy with ANB reductions of 2 to 2.5^{o}.

- There is an acceleration of expected mandibular corpus length increase by approximately 1 to 1.5mm a year during the period of active appliance wear.

- The lower anterior face height as a percentage of total face height increases by approximately 2%.

- The expected average linear growth of lower face height, anteriorly and posteriorly, appears to double.

- The upper incisors erupt a little and upright by 10-12°, (ie never activate the labial bow).

- In Design Card 1 the lower incisors procline by 5° (range - 2 to +14°), figures are not yet available for the capped FR (Design Card 2).

- The most retroclined lower incisors at the start of treatment procline most and the most proclined lower incisors at the start of treatment procline least, ie the Class II Frankel can be used in the treatment of Skeletal II bimaxillary protrusions.

- There is substantial dentoalveolar change superimposed on a small but useful skeletal change.

- The appliances appear to have a good effect on the circumoral musculature (not measurable) and 'soften' Class II Division 2 types of lip activity.

- The capped FR is useful in the treatment of both deep bite Class II Division 1 malocclusion and Class II Division 2 malocclusion which is first converted to Class II Division 1 and then put into the Class II displacement functional appliance (either a capped FR or a medium opening activator).

CLINICAL : LABORATORY INTERFACE

The Class II Frankel is a 'difficult to tolerate' appliance which must be made and presented to the patient with discretion and care. There is NO need to trim the working casts in the buccal shield area. Buccal shield wax relief wants to be less, rather than more (see Design Cards 1 and 2 for details). Do NOT disc teeth on the working cast ie E|E or D|D to settle the palatal wires between the teeth. The thicker wires prescribed are recommended for appliance rigidity and stability. The lower labial vestibule should be vertically stretched to a **moderate** extent during the lower impression. 1 in 2 patients cannot tolerate deep lower labial pelotes.

PATIENT INSTRUCTIONS FOR THE CLASS II FRANKEL APPLIANCE - Design Cards 1 and 2

The appliance is essentially a DAYTIME and also a night-time appliance. **Over a 2-3 month** period the patient should **build up 18 - 20 hours of FR wear.** There are two rules:

1. The appliance MUST, whenever it is removed from the mouth, **be placed into its box,** where it will be safe from family pets, waiters, school friends, etc.

2. The patient MUST learn **to speak WITH THE TEETH HELD TOGETHER** whilst moving the lips well and learn NOT to bounce the appliance up and down while speaking or resting. Children should be encouraged to read to their parents each evening during the first month of appliance wear.

The patient should **start off by wearing the appliance during the day only.** After 2-3 weeks, when they will have built up 5-6 hours wear per day, they should start to wear the appliance at night. If the appliance falls out at night, it is not being worn enough during the day to establish the necessary subconscious reflexes.

For Design Card 1 routinely check the lingual of the lower incisors for soreness or abrasion.

If the patient cannot settle into the Class II Frankel well and good progress is not being made by 4-5 months, consider switching to a medium opening activator - palatal (Design Card 8A).

REACTIVATION OF THE CLASS II FRANKEL APPLIANCE

Dependent on the initial activation and how rapidly the patient has settled, the Frankel appliance will become inactive at 3-5 months. At this point the appliance should be reactivated. A completely horizontal cut is made from the mesial of the buccal shield for 8-10mm into the shield, parallel to the occlusal plane and just above the lingual hanger wire. The cut then turns through 90° and travels vertically to the bottom of the shield avoiding 'nicking' the flattened horizontal part of the hanger wire. The cut should be 2-3mm distal to the vertical part of the lingual hanger wire. The lingual hanger assembly and lower labial pelotes are thus mesial to the reversed 'L' shaped cut (see page 19). A wax knife is then put into the vertical cut and **gently** twisted to give a 1.5-2mm advance. Measure this from the movement of the free flattened end of the hanger wire. Each FR appliance should be advanced 1-3 times in SMALL increments.

PRESCRIPTION FOR THE CLASS III FRANKEL -
Design Card 3

This atlas is devoted to the treatment of Class II malocclusion. The Class III Frankel is however described, both for the sake of completeness in illustrating the Frankel systems, but also for the light that it sheds on a 'Functional Component Analysis Approach to appliance design.' **The Class III Frankel** (Design Card 3) is used in the management of Class III occlusions in the **early** mixed dentition with reverse overjets, mild to moderate Class III overbites on a mild Skeletal III pattern with average to low FMPA's. The appliance is not appropriate for the long faced Class III nor for the older patient. The response to the appliance may be slow and it does need advance of the upper labial pelotes at 4-5 months. The occlusal improvement may 'stick' at approximately 9 months and a remake should be considered. Usage of this appliance at Kingston has never reached a substantial level and a usually preferred alternative is a customised facemask or headgear to a lower en-masse plate. The use of headgear to the lower arch was described by Orton, Sullivan, Battagel & Orton in the *B. J. Orthod.* 10: 2-12, 1983.

The appliance works in a reverse fashion to the Class II Frankel.

- The lower arch is totally constrained labially, buccally and vertically.

- The upper arch is free to erupt vertically, buccally and labially.

- The mandible develops vertically with slight backward hinging.

- The maxillary complex moves forwards a little with slight improvement of SNA ($1-2^o$) and towards a positive value of ANB. ANB values invariably remain in the low Skeletal III tendency range.

- The lower incisors retrocline $5-10^o$ and surprisingly upper incisors retrocline as well $3-4^o$. The appliance is therefore useful for treating a bimaxillary protrusion on a Skeletal III base.

PATIENT INSTRUCTIONS FOR THE CLASS III FRANKEL

These are identical to the Class II Frankel.

THE CLINICAL USEFULNESS OF THE FRANKEL SYSTEMS

Prior to the seventies the Frankel systems were relatively unknown in the United Kingdom, they began to be widely used in the seventies and early eighties. After an initial trial many clinicians ceased to use the appliances on the grounds that the failure rate did not warrant the effort. The system is very 'technician sensitive' and many indifferently made Frankel appliances have been seen. Provided the clinician follows the guidance that is outlined and appliances are made that are **mildly active,** look fairly comfortable and generally improve the patient's facial appearance; **then** this can be an elegant appliance system. If the patient looks grossly facially distended, then it may be the wrong system for the patient, have an over-active bite or be poorly made. The Class II Frankel is probably appropriate to 20% of Skeletal II malocclusion and the Class III Frankel to 10% of Skeletal III problems. Whilst these systems have a lesser place in the functional appliance armamentarium, they are described first because of their historical importance and the neat way that they display the principles of a functional component analysis.

FURTHER READING and REFERENCES - See Chapter Six

Clinical guidance on prescription

- **Prescribe for Class II Division 1 occlusions with, average FMPA, normal to reduced overbite, mild to moderate skeletal discrepancy, relatively aligned arches, and with profile retrognathia.**

- Complete the design card. The main modification may be the wire arrangement on the lingual of 321|123 if there should be imbrication of teeth in the lower labial segment; a single wire can be used on 21|12 only.

- **The bite technique.** First practice the patient in the bite you want. Then use a gas flame and warm a sheet of wax and form a small roll of a non-brittle wax eg Tenatex. **Use too little rather than too much, as large wax overhangs tend to inaccuracy,** since you cannot see clearly what you are doing. Get the patient to **close slowly, hold;** and **stay there. Take the bite out of the mouth, chill it** and **retry it.** Then cut out a small window for $\frac{1|1}{1|1}$ and $\frac{5|}{5|}$ region to check the centreline and buccal opening. The bite material should be wax and we do not recommend silicone bites due to rebound in thick sections.

- **The bite objectives.** Approximately 4-5mm forward and 2-2.5mm open in the premolar region. Reduce the activation for the small and timid patient. It is better to take an under active bite and have the patient accept the appliance since the Frankel can easily be advanced at 10-12 weeks.

- **Impression tray choice.** Choose perforated impression trays which are a close rather than a generous fit. Choose deepish rather than shallow trays. The intention is to gently stretch the vestibular reflection **vertically** and avoid flattening it buccally with too wide a tray. Use the sticky, stiff, white strip wax as supplied by Modern Materials to modify the rim of a standard Coe impresssion tray.

- **The upper impression tray.** Add a peripheral roll in the 654|456 region and on the posterior edge of the tray. Lift the lips and cheeks when seating the tray as completely as possible. Then stretch the cheeks vertically.

- **The lower impression tray.** Add a strip of wax on the heels of the tray and extend buccal to 6|6 .**Add a lingual strip in the 3+3 region.** The metal of the tray must not bottom out of the alginate lingual to the lower labial segment, as mucosal rubbing is a potent source of patient difficulty. Finally take a double roll of white wax and add it on the **inside of the tray** on the labial of 3+3 with vertical extension of the rim. Seat the tray fully and stretch the lip vertically, not outwards.

Technical guidance on construction

- Rinse and dry the impressions, and cast them in a mixture of 50% stone and 50% plaster.

- **Do not trim the impression periphery** on the buccal, and maintain the sulcus reflection in full. The acrylic will be finished into this reflection. Buccal shield and labial pelote extension is determined by the clinician's impression technique, rather than by an arbitrary trimming of the model.

- See that the models will settle easily into the bite. This is why the clinician should chill his bite and retry it.

- Articulate the models on a plain line or plasterless articulator with the articulation from the **back** of the working models.

- At this point dismount the articulation, look at the models held in a maximum intercuspation bite (ie where the patient has started from) and check that the forward open bite is within the limits outlined above. If the bite is too forward, too open, lopsided or the centrelines are significantly off, then contact the clinician before proceeding.

- Complete the lingual portion and the lower labial pelotes in auto-polymerised resin, finish and highly polish.

- Wax out for the upper and lower buccal shields. There should be a 'comfort wash' at the periphery of the buccal shields, with 1.0mm of wax at the lower buccal gingival margins; 2mm of upper buccal crown relief is required.

- Assemble the lingual portion and labial pelotes and complete the wirework prior to joining the upper to the lower. The lower should be joined to the upper with no occlusal line constraint. **Particularly for the small and timid patient buccal waxing relief should be kept to a minimum.**

- The finished buccal shields should be slim, highly polished, non-porous and have a rounded slightly beaded margin.

- The following are the size (in mm) and function of the wires. The clearance between the wires and buccal shield waxing is 0.75mm.

Lower incisor guide wires	0.7 minimises eruption of lower incisors but may induce proclination.
Lower pelote wire	0.9 connection between lower pelotes and shields.
Lower lingual hanger	1.5 to support the lower lingual guidance flange & for advancement. The wire ends should be flattened and parallel to the occlusal plane.
Anterior palatal wire	1.0 to support the FR vertically, minimise palatal tipping of 21|12 , maintain a rounded out 21|12 & to act as a Cl II traction force on 4|4 .
Transpalatal wire	1.125 for lateral stability, Cl II traction force on 6|6 , reduction of eruption but not as a buccal check to 6|6 (no interdental trimming to seat the wire).
Labial arch 21|12	1.0 to provide a labial restraint of 21|12 with minimal tipping.

Functional Component Objectives

1. Sagittal restraint of the maxillary dentition.
2. Some vertical restraint of the maxilla and maxillary dentition.
3. Freedom for buccal movement of the upper buccal segments.
4. No **vertical** constraint to lower buccal segment eruption.
5. Limitation of buccal movement of lower cheek teeth.
6. Maximised increments of the condylar growth mechanism.
7. Minimised uprighting of the upper incisors (average 10°).
8. Minimised proclination of the lower incisors (average 5°).
9. A relaxed lips together seal, without conscious effort, at the end of retention.

NOTE This last objective is rarely fully present at the end of the active phase of treatment, but may slowly develop during a protracted retention period of diminished wearing of the appliance.

10. Some unfurling of the labio-mental fold.
11. A Class I incisal relationship with a reduced overjet and a reduced but complete overbite.

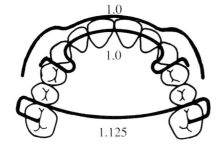

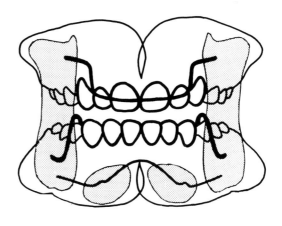

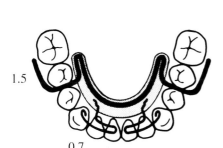

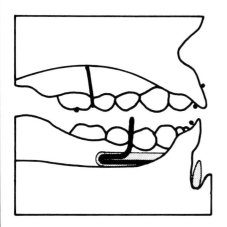

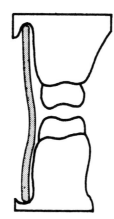

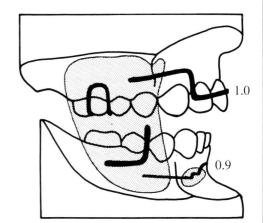

Wire size conversion (mm to American Gauge) : 0.7 = 21, 0.9 = 19, 1.0 = 18, 1.125 = 17, 1.5 = 15

A FRANKEL APPLIANCE with
LOWER INCISAL CAPPING for Class II Division 1
occlusions with deep and complete overbites

2

Clinical guidance on prescription

- **Prescribe for Class II Division 1 occlusions with, average to low FMPA, increased or deep and complete overbites, with mild to moderate skeletal discrepancy, relatively aligned arches, and with profile retrognathia.**

- Complete the design card. The capped Frankel is slightly more of a mouthful than the standard Frankel. Confirm that you feel that the patient can support this appliance. The capped Frankel now forms 50% of the Frankel appliances prescribed at Kingston Hospital.

- Pay particular attention to mild irregularity in 3+3 region and be prepared to specify any finger plastering that is needed to permit alignment within the labial segment capping. The acrylic must maintain contact with the incisal edges and particularly with the lingual surfaces of most of the lower incisors.

- **The bite technique.** Similar to Design Card 1.

- **The bite objectives.** Approximately 5mm forward, open by 3-3.5mm in the premolar region. Reduce the bite activation for the small and timid patient, and **also** reduce the buccal shield relief.

- **Impression technique.** Similar to Design Card 1, but be prepared to go for a little more vertical stretching of the vestibule on the labial of 321|123 . If the lower impression tray bottoms out on the lingual of 3+3 it will give a pressure sore area.

- On all Class II Frankels check that the flattened end of the lingual flange wire is bilaterally symmetric and **parallel to the buccal occlusal plane** to permit easy reactivation of the appliance.

- Advance the appliance at 3-4 months and again at 6-8 months. Do not worry if the bite is opened by 21|12 occluding with the lower capping, since overbite reduction is a major treatment aim.

Technical guidance on construction

- The casting, trimming, articulation and bite checking are similar to Design Card 1.

- Check the need for any light plastering on 321|123 lingually and labially if there is spacing or rotation, to permit alignment within the capping. Do not cover the lingual surfaces of most of the lower incisors with plaster. There **must not be a baggy fit** of the capping on the lower labial segment.

- Buccal waxing is similar to Design Card 1. Minimise the buccal relief if in doubt.

- Bend the wires for the lower lingual hanger and the lower labial pelotes.

- Sheet wax is laid around the required area on the lower lingual segment and the pre-bent hanger is set into the wax.

- This assembly is lifted off, a cast made of the fitting surface, the wax boiled off and replaced with autopolymerising acrylic.

- The lower labial pelotes will have been constructed on the lower cast using wax dams and autopolymerising resin.

- Both the lingual hanger assembly and the labial pelotes should be **highly polished** before being sealed into place. The plastering and construction of the shaped wax sheet should ensure a close but smooth internal surface of the capping.

- Wire sizes (in mm) are :

Lower pelote wire	0.9 connection between lower pelotes and shields.
Lower lingual hanger	1.5 to support the lower labial segment capping & for advancement.
Anterior palatal wire	1.0 to support the FR vertically, minimise palatal tipping of 21|12 , maintain a rounded out 21|12 & as a Cl II traction force on 4|4 .
Transpalatal wire	1.125 for lateral stability, Cl II traction force on 6|6 , reduction of eruption but **not** as a buccal stop to 6|6 (no interdental trimming to seat the wire).
Labial arch 21|12	1.0 to provide a Cl II restraint of 21|12 with minimal tipping.

- The buccal wax shield relief should be smoothed and polished to gain the smoothest possible inner surface to the shields. Care should be exercised where the upper and lower models are joined.

- Wax dams can be placed at the mesial and distal border of the buccal shields to restrict acrylic flow to the required area. The acrylic is applied to both sides of the appliance and cured in the pressure vessel. The aim is thin, strong, dense, buccal shields with well rounded edges.

- **See page 15 for advice on reactivation of the FR.**

A FRANKEL APPLIANCE with
LOWER INCISAL CAPPING for Class II Division 1
occlusions with deep and complete overbites

FUNCTIONAL
APPLIANCE   **2**
DESIGN CARD

Functional Component Objectives

1-11 Same as DESIGN CARD NO.1.

12. Good vertical control of the lower labial segment.

13. To flatten an increased lower curve of Spee.

14. To maximise the increase in anterior and posterior lower face height and to increase the proportion of lower face height to total face height.

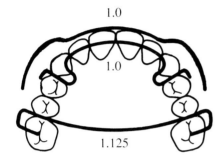

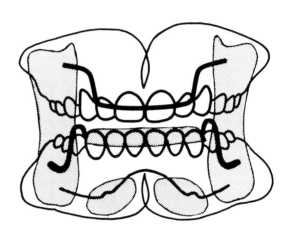

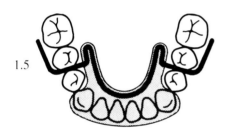

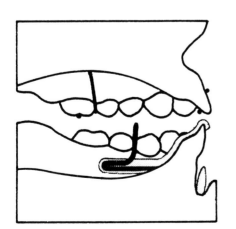

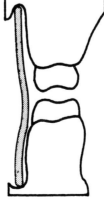

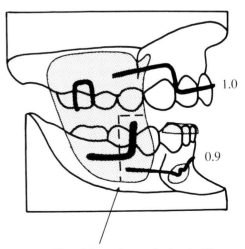

Line of the cut for reactivating the FR at 3-5 months ; see page 15.

Wire size conversion (mm to American Gauge) : 0.9 = 19, 1.0 = 18, 1.125 = 17, 1.5 = 15

Clinical guidance on prescription

- **Prescribe for Class III occlusions with, average to low FMPA, aligned arches, bimaxillary proclination, a mild to moderate skeletal III base, who are in the early mixed dentition, and have facial maxillary flatness.**

- Whilst older patients, with slightly longer faces, more crowding and more skeletal prognathia can be treated with the FR3 appliance, it is best employed in the **early mixed dentition** for the case type outlined above.

- Complete the design card. The transpalatal wire must be distal to the maxillary terminal molar. The lower buccal segment teeth all need a vertical occlusal stop. Full lower sulcus shield extension makes the skeletal III patient look even more prognathic. The non-functional lower part of the buccal shield has been removed, leaving the lower edge of the shield 2-3mm below the lower buccal gingival margins.

- **The bite** should be hinged downwards enough to clear the incisal overbite, with the mandible as far retruded as possible.

- **The upper impression.** Choose a deep tray that is not too wide and will not stretch the mucosal reflection laterally and flatten it. Take two rolls of white stiffened rim wax and mould these to the **inside** of the tray, extending the margin vertically by 4-5mm. Warn the patient that seating the tray will be uncomfortable, then try it in the mouth. Don't overload the tray, use an alginate mix that will flow well and seat the tray **fully** without muscle trimming.

- **The lower impression.** No special features.

- **Patient instructions.** Similar to the Class II Frankel. Learn to speak without moving the lower jaw, holding the teeth together. 18-20 hours wear per day. Keep the appliance in its box when out of the mouth.

- Enthusiastic 8-9 year olds who take to the FR3, do so very readily and frequently show rapid initial changes which may then appear to stick. At the 3-5 month point **advance** the upper labial pelotes.

- Watch that the pelote advance does not destabilise the appliance.

- Remake at 9-12 months and continue nocturnal retention for 1-2 years.

Technical guidance on construction

- The casting, trimming, articulation and bite checking are similar to Design Card 1.

- The upper labial pelotes are constructed to a smooth and highly polished state ready to be positioned when the upper cast has been waxed out.

- The labial surface of $\overline{321|123}$ should be marked with a pencil halfway between the incisal tip and gingival margin. A half round groove should be cut along this line using a fine round file so that the lower labial bow of 1.25mm wire will gently nestle 1/3 of its thickness into this groove.

- **Buccal waxing.** The lower has a 'comfort wash' of wax. The upper has 2.5mm of crown relief and 1.5mm on the buccal mucosa and for sulcus relief. At the full depth of the impression, where there is forced vertical extension of the vestibule, the wax relief should be reduced so that the beaded upper edge of the buccal shield will stretch the vestibule well. The buccal wax must be smoothed and hand polished before sealing in the wires and the upper labial pelotes.

- Wire sizes (in mm) are :

Upper pelote wire	0.9 connection between upper pelotes and shields. This wire should have straight ends allowing the pelotes to be advanced at a later stage.
Anterior palatal wire	1.0 passive labial guidance of $21|12$.
Transpalatal wire	1.125 distal to the terminal molar and in hard contact at gingival level.
Lower labial bow	1.25 labial constraint of $\overline{321|123}$.
Lower occlusal wire	1.0 vertical stop to the lower buccal teeth.

- There should be 0.75mm clearance between the buccal wax and the wire to allow an easy acrylic flow and retention of the wires in the plastic.

- Wax dams can be placed for the buccal shields. The acrylic is applied to both sides of the appliance and cured in the pressure vessel.

- The acrylic should be dense, polished, thin but with well rounded edges. The edges of all shields should be well rounded with no taper.

Functional Component Objectives

1. Total occlusal, buccal and labial **restraint** of the **mandibular dentition.**
2. Total **freedom** of the **maxillary dentition** to erupt outwards and downwards.
3. Mild downwards and backwards hinging of the mandible with sagittal arrest of the shadow of the symphysis.
4. Forward development of 'A' point.
5. Lateral expansion of the maxillary buccal dentition.
6. Lateral constraint of the mandibular buccal dentition.
7. Lingual uprighting of the lower incisors.
8. Mild palatal uprighting of the upper incisors ie minimised proclination where III are already procumbent.
9. The overall induction of a Class I incisal relationship with a tendency to an increased positive overjet and increased overbite.

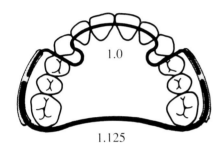

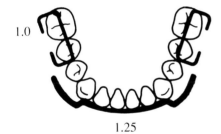

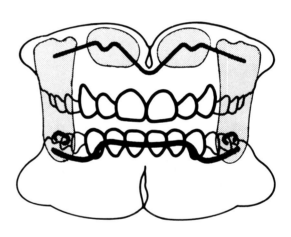

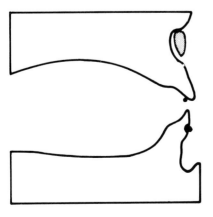

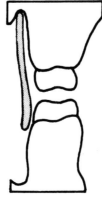

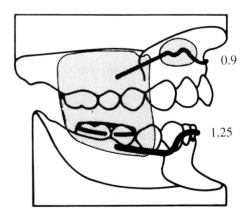

Wire size conversion (mm to American Gauge) : 0.9 = 19, 1.0 = 18, 1.125 = 17, 1.25 = 16

CHAPTER TWO

EXPANSION AND LABIAL SEGMENT ALIGNMENT APPLIANCES (ELSAA's) DESIGN CARDS 4 - 7

In the sagittal correction of a Class II Division 1 occlusion some transverse expansion of the maxillary dentition is commonly required. This can be confirmed by getting the patient to hold their mandible forward into a corrected Class I incisal position when a crossbite tendency in the buccal segments is usually apparent. Also, many patients who would benefit facially from functional appliances have moderate to severe labial segment crowding. Functional appliances of the activator type traditionally required a relatively aligned upper labial segment, and were historically designed to be used in cases without substantial lower labial segment crowding. Instanding and malaligned teeth will limit the amount of forward displacement that can be obtained in the functional treatment to improve the patient's retrognathia. Additionally, upper incisors retrocline 10-12° during the functional phase of treatment and therefore need to be at approximately 120-125° to the maxillary plane at the start of the functional phase of treatment.

A range of removable appliances has evolved which will allow these problems to be solved in the mixed or permanent dentition. We are indebted to John Mew and his Mew 1 appliance for initiating this section of our clinical work. Practitioners need to cope with the paradox that upper labial segment crowding in Class II Division 2 and some Class II Division 1 occlusions provides welcome tooth substance for full upper labial segment arch alignment, initial palatal root torquing of <u>111</u> and maxillary anchorage creation; ie the overjets are frequently increased prior to the functional phase of treatment. A sports guard should be provided during this phase of treatment.

The Kingston Medium Opening Activator (MOA) has clasps to help retain the appliance in place and assist the patient to accept the appliance with confidence. These simple activators have worked well for many, many practitioners. The standard tooth borne functional appliance such as, the Andresen activator, is on average less well tolerated but has buccal segment acrylic that can be shaped to contact the teeth so that their eruption is guided buccally by the facets. In this manner the eruption of the buccal segment teeth can be influenced towards a wider lateral arch dimension. If the practitioner is going to seek the benefits of a **clasped activator**, then maxillary expansion (4-5 mm on <u>6+6</u>) needs to be undertaken with an ELSAA prior to the functional appliance phase. Modern steel screws are very efficient and should be expanded 2 x 1/4 turns per week, or alternatively **1/8 turn per day.** The key to success is **well made** and **well adjusted** cribs. The technician should consult Adams's textbook for the detail of construction. **Each treatment visit** the clinician should first **check the cribbing** since unless this is highly retentive the system cannot work. Screws should be routinely replaced when they are 4/5ths extended and later fused when the appropriate expansion is achieved. Stop short of going into buccal crossbite (X-bite) and, if there is a risk of this, add a palatal acrylic shelf to prevent a buccal overbite developing. If the child has any wire or acrylic fracture they must not leave out the appliance, but should bring it back in their mouths for immediate repair on the clinician's or technician's premises. The expansion achieved is unstable until approximately 4-6 months into the functional phase of treatment. In the first 4-6 months of functional treatment, the previous fused ELSAA **must** be worn for all meals and whenever the functional appliance is out of the mouth. The ELSAA is kept in the patient's functional appliance box. The expansion achieved with these removable appliances is simply done compared to a hyrax screw, can easily achieve a centimetre of maxillary expansion if required (it rarely is), and induces less buccal tipping than quadhelix cemented appliances.

The anterior palatal wires are either stiff and rely on the screw as much as activation for nudging the incisors into alignment, or are long recurved wires without coils relying on length for spring flexibility and wire thickness to avoid deformation. Most wires are unboxed and unguarded and reasonably well tolerated by patients. They give few occlusal problems. Labial bows are less commonly used now than previously. It must be remembered that a labial bow will tighten as the screw is expanded. **A labial bow should be tested for contact pressure with the incisors and eased**

forward just out of contact each visit. The pressure is best tested by tapping the labial bow with the handle of a mouth mirror. The pressure of the wire on the tooth is revealed by the pitch of the note made when the mirror handle taps the bow. The higher the 'ping', the more the pressure, ie no note, no pressure. Excessive prolonged pressure of the labial bow on ⊥⊥⊥ induced by a remorseless expansion of the midline screw can cause pulpal death.

Acrylic is generally saddled (Design Cards 4, 5, 7), but may less commonly be a full palate (Design Card 6). Heat cured appliances are preferred.

PRESCRIPTION   TECHNIQUE

The clinician should spend time sitting at the patient's side thinking what he wishes this simple but powerful appliance system to achieve. A dento-alveolar component analysis is undertaken and the clinician then assembles the appliance components, including retention, expansion, labial alignment and acrylic, to design an ELSAA that is appropriate to the patient's particular problem. It may be convenient to add a few anterior brackets to close mesio-distal spacing. It is important to prevent spacing opening in the labial segment, whilst the incisors are proclined and aligned and an anterior sectional archwire 3+3 or 4+4 may be appropriate. It is also important to avoid spending too much of the precious first treatment year in the ELSAA. The patient's cooperation is highest initially and one wants to take maximum advantage of this for the more demanding functional appliance. Treatment times for ELSAA's for Class II Division 1 should only be about 3-4 months and for Class II Division 2 conversion slightly longer, perhaps 6 months.

CLINICAL CHECKPOINTS WITH THE ELSAA

- **First check the cribbing** (ie the Adams's clasps).

- Learn the skills of putting each retentive arrowhead where it will work best.

- Make sure that the patient is **fully** seating the appliance, especially after expanding the screw.

- Check that the screw **is working** either by looking at the expected midline opening, or more tediously, counting the turns since the last visit.

- The average screw will reach 4/5ths of its travel by the 3rd appointment; **automatically replace it** at this point.

- If the expected expansion is not achieved, is it the patient or your instructions, is the plate not being seated firmly, or is the spindle of the screw loose (1 patient in 25) ?

- Check that the anterior wires are giving the precise labial alignment needed; if not, adjust, modify or replace the palatal wires.

- Test the labial bow for pressure on 21|12 and ensure that it is a passive, rather than an active, guide wire.

- During the active phase of treatment the ELSAA appliance should be worn FULLTIME, INCLUDING MEALS. This implies minimising 'snacking' between meals and regular tooth, palate and appliance brushing after each meal.

- When the desired lateral expansion of the upper buccal segments has been achieved, **seal the midline screw with acrylic.**

- Ensure that this ELSAA phase of treatment is completed in closer to 3 rather than 6 months.

FURTHER READING and REFERENCES - See Chapter Six

Clinical guidance on prescription

- **Prescribe for any Class II Division 1 occlusions to be treated by a clasped activator (Design Cards 8-11) or intrusion appliances (15-17) where a sagittal change in the arch relationship requires expansion of the upper buccal segments and alignment of the upper labial segment.**

- Design the appliance by undertaking a quiet, contemplative analysis of individual erupted (and unerupted) misplaced teeth and then decide **what is needed** (not necessarily ideally required) to enter the sagittal phase of arch correction.

- The objective is to get into the functional appliance rapidly (3-4 months).

- The component analysis of the appliances should in order be:
  1. **Appliance retention.** Which teeth to clasp and where. Tailor the pattern of clasping to fit in with the other wirework.
  2. **Occlusal support.** Tooth rests and acrylic coverage.
  3. **Palato-labial segment components.** This will relate to the pattern of anterior crowding and may be wires or acrylic only plus the effect of the screw.
  4. **Labial components.** Either none, a labial bow, or some anterior brackets.
  5. **The acrylic.** This should contact 65|56 only, 654|456 , or be a full palate.
  6. **The expansion screw.** Is symmetric expansion needed, or does there need to be an individual spring on an instanding buccal segment tooth (eg Design Card 7 iv)? Expand 1/8 of a turn per day or two 1/4 turns per week.

Design 4 i. This Elsaa design is most commonly prescribed. The labial bow is adjusted to be out of contact with 1|1 and is provided to act as a **guide** for incisor alignment and **not** as a retraction bow.

Design 4 ii. The palatal wires require more skill to adjust but can be useful in the alignment of the more instanding 2|2 (see also 5 iii and 5 iv).

Design 4 iii. If incisor alignment is slow, (decide this by the 2nd visit), or looks difficult, possibly due to rotations or to acute space shortage for 2, then bond brackets anteriorly on 21|12 , 321|123 or 4321|1234 and use nickel titanium aligning wires with space opening push coils as needed.

Design 4 iv. As for 4 iii, but gives more flexibility on the palatal activation of instanding 2|2 .

Technical guidance on construction

- Rinse and dry the impression and cast in a mixture of 50% stone and 50% plaster.

- Try to have the study models available if possible and try to undertstand the detail of the clinician's intention.

- If there is doubt a telephone call is appropriate at this stage.

- The 0.8mm double crib on 65 works extremely well, when made well. But it is difficult to adjust when made poorly. Place any small steps needed in the bridge of the crib to keep the bridge wire close to the buccal surface of 65.

- The butterfly occlusal rest is made from a 1.0mm cross type clasp made by Krupp for wrought denture clasps.

- The palatal wires should be bent in smooth, rounded curves. The stiff wires (0.9mm) must have enough overlap to accomodate the opening of the screw. The more flexible wires (0.8mm) must have 3-4 mm of **spare wire at the end of the spring** to allow for tooth movement and expansion.

- If a labial wire is present it should be bent into a smooth ideal curve and permit 2-3mm of 3|3 expansion.

- Mesio-distal acrylic placement needs to be precise and follow the clinical guidance.

- The midline thickness of the screw and acrylic should be **no more than 5.0mm to maximise patient tolerance.** (Clinicians should reject overthick plates).

- With the very deeply vaulted palate, some plastering of the depth of the vault may be appropriate.

- **Heat cured semi-transparent acrylic is preferred.** If an autopolymerised resin is used, it must be a high quality resin that is hard and will take and keep a high polish.

Functional Component Objectives

1. Rapid maxillary arch alignment prior to functional therapy (3-4 months).

2. Rounding out of the upper labial segment :

   a) Increasing the inter-canine width (2-2.5mm).

   b) Reducing upper incisor crowding by proclination (125° to the Maxillary Plane) and providing anchorage for the functional appliance Class II displacement phase of treatment.

   This is achieved by the use of palatal wires, the labial wire and/or labial brackets as necessary.

3. Lateral expansion of upper first molars (4-5mm) and a premolar width sufficient to accomodate the forward translation of the mandibular arch. Do not expand into a bilateral total crossbite; if there is a risk of this add a small shelf of acrylic palatal to the upper buccal segments.

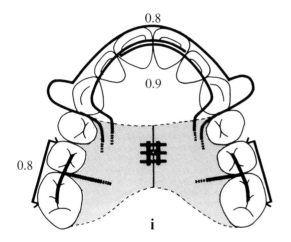

i

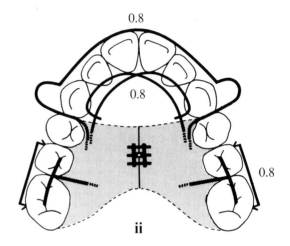

ii

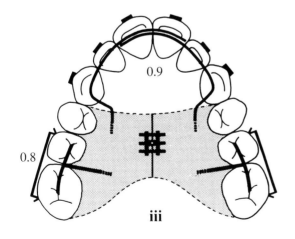

iii

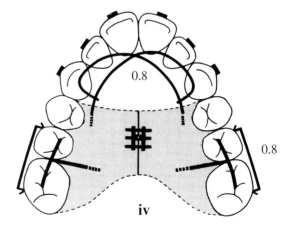

iv

Wire size conversion (mm to American Gauge) : 0.8 = 20, 0.9 = 19

Clinical guidance on prescription

- **Prescribe Designs 5 i & 5 ii for any Class II Division 2 occlusions of moderate to severe extent.** This type of occlusion should be converted from Division 2 to Division 1, and then treated with an activator (Design Card 8A) or a capped Frankel (Design Card 2). **Avoid extraction of upper premolars even in the presence of severe upper arch crowding.** The accomodation of maxillary crowding with this approach is dramatic. The lingual stabilisation of $\overline{3211123}$ with a medium opening activator (Design Card 8A) **allows lower mid-arch extractions and the use of lower fixed appliances within the functional phase of treatment without retroclination of** $\overline{3211123}$.

- **Prescribe Designs 5 iii & 5 iv for any Class II Division 1 malocclusion with significantly instanding 2|2 and moderately crowded upper labial segment.** Add brackets to the upper labial segment as appropriate, as in Designs 4 iii & 4 iv.

- General design features as for Design Card 4.

Design 5 i. This is a most useful design for a classical Class II Division 2 incisor presentation. Ignore the anterior crowding and 2|2 labially trapped position, since the posterior expansion, posterior distallisation of upper buccal segments and labial movement of 1|1 will take care of this. The 0.8mm spring on 1|1 should be activated labially and **gingivally** to induce protrusion and **intrusion** of 1|1. Ignore any difficulty with the incisor occlusion, the patient will adapt to this. The ELSAA's for Class II Division 2 occlusions can be used for intrusion on 1|1 or 21|12 . The spring is activated gingivally as well as labially **to raise 1|1 above the functioning level of the lower lip-line during expressive behaviour.** This also helps the 'gummy Class II Div 2' patient. Be prepared to use **two** ELSAA's in the more severe Class II Division 2 cases. First use Design 5 i, followed by Design 5 ii as the incisors progressively align.

Design 5 ii. The spring on 1|1 in 5 i will exhaust in 3-4 visits. For the moderate to severe case remake the ELSAA on a 1-2 week appliance turn around to continue the alignment. If 4| or 4|4 tend to crossbite, recognise this in the pattern of the cribbing chosen and **relieve the acrylic palatal to the upper first premolars.**

Design 5 iii. Make sure that there is sufficient length of wire to continue to reach the distal of 2|2 in the presence of 3-4mm of midline screw expansion without having to radically rework the spring.

Design 5 iv. Similarly for 3|3 . As the springs become larger use 1.0mm wire rather than 0.9mm. Consider supplementing with anterior brackets as in Designs 4 iii & 4 iv if there is slowness in aligning 2|2 .

Technical guidance on construction

- The casting of the model, understanding of the design, crib, screw and acrylic work is similar to Design Card 4 .

- The palatal wires are more complex. They should appear symmetric in form and follow a natural curve without adapting to individual tooth misplacement. The irregularity of teeth will rapidly disappear as the spring is activated.

- The palatal wire must closely follow the palatal slope of the incisors and the anterior palate to minimise occlusal discomfort for the patient.

- The rapidity of alignment means that the technician **must appreciate the requirements of the spring after 3-4 activations.** The central incisors will have moved forwards 4-5 millimetres and will be on a broader curve. There must be sufficient recurve in the wire to permit the advancement and particularly sufficient length in the anterior part of the wire to accomodate the increased arc of the incisors. A rule of thumb is to extend the anterior part (the pushing portion) 1-1.5mm past the true distal of the teeth being moved labially ie either 1|1 or 21|12 .

- The length of the wire gives it flexibility. Coils are not needed.

- The thickness of the wire 0.8mm, 0.9mm or 1.0mm gives the wire stability and resistance to deformation & damage.

- Wires must not be overworked in construction.

- Where acrylic is to be relieved from 4| then the tag end of the adjacent crib must be contoured away to permit the easing of the acrylic without damaging the wire.

Functional Component Objectives

1. Arch alignment prior to functional therapy (may take up to 6 months) in these types of cases.

2. Rounding out of the upper labial segment :

    a) Proclination of retroclined 1|1 to 125° to the maxillary plane in Class II Division 2 cases (Designs i & ii).

    b) Alignment of instanding 2|2 (Designs iii & iv).

    c) Reducing incisor crowding by proclination.

    d) Increasing intercanine width (Designs iii & iv).

3. The generation of maxillary labial segment anchorage for use during the Class II functional phase of treatment.

4. Lateral expansion of molar and premolar width, but beware over expansion of 4|4 in Class II Division 2 cases when 4|4 are in an existing buccal crossbite. In these cases relieve palatal to 4|4 on the baseplate.

5. To torque 1|1 apices palatally in Class II Division 2 cases.

6. To raise the level of the incisal tips of 1|1 so that the lower lip functions BELOW them during **expressive behaviour** in Class II Division 2 cases.

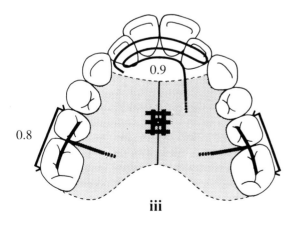

i

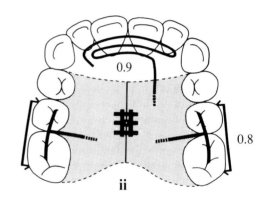

ii

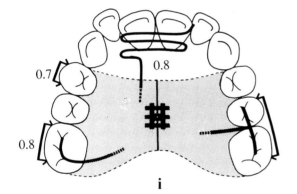

iii

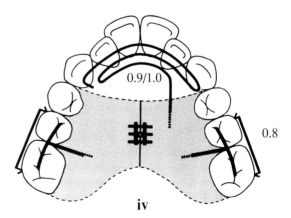

iv

Wire size conversion (mm to American Gauge) : 0.7 = 21, 0..8 = 20, 0.9 = 19, 1.0 = 18.

Clinical guidance on prescription

- Designs 6 i & 6 ii can be prescribed for any **deep bite** Class II Division 1 occlusions with only **mild insetting** of 2|2 and **the need for moderate to marked expansion of the upper buccal segments.**

- Designs 6 iii & 6 iv can be used for a deep-bite Class II Division 2 case in which the clinician is concerned about incisal mucosal trauma or damage to the palatal spring. In general this design is less satisfactory than the simpler designs shown in 5 i & 5 ii.

- Designs 6 i & 6 ii have been surprisingly useful for quite deep-bite Class II Division 1 cases, in which the main anterior problem has been a broadening and rounding out of the upper arch.

- The height, depth and hardness of the anterior bite-plate are key technical features. The trimming should be undertaken very precisely by the clinician.

- To obtain a well made appliance, take **both** upper and lower working impressions, ask the technician to articulate on a plane line articulator and open the hinge to provide a moderate (but not excessive) anterior flat bite-plate of the height requested.

- It is strongly recommended that **the appliance is constructed in heat cured acrylic.**

- The acrylic trimming should be undertaken with care (see 6 ii, iii & iv). First use an acrylic bur held obliquely on the palatal fit surface of the plate, **do not** trim the occlusal. When the acrylic in the incisal and canine regions has been undermined appropriately then use a soft white rubber wheel from the polished side of the acrylic to round the bite-plate into an ideal curve that contacts the instanding teeth only.

- **Expansion.** The midline screw should be turned 1/8 of a turn per day for optimal effect. CAUTION; this rate of expansion **only works in the presence of highly retentive clasping** and the patient should be seen at least every 4 weeks to check this.

- If a rebuild of the anterior bite-plate is needed, then a wax squash bite should be taken over the labial segment tips of teeth and the anterior palate of the plate. A laboratory rebuild in pressure set auto-polymerising resin will be more accurate and harder than an intra-oral quick cure-resin application.

- Designs 6 iii & 6 iv require moderately thick anterior bite-plates (which may give tolerance problems) in order to reduce the frequent acrylic fractures that occur as a consequence of boxing out the springs.

Technical guidance on construction

- Encourage the clinician to provide a lower working impression or model and articulate on a plane line articulator. Unless precise guidance has been given, open the bite enough to provide a moderate anterior bite-plate ie 3/5ths of the way up the palatal of 1 from the gingival margin.

- Prepare the wire work.

- Choose a screw that in width will fit reasonably into the vault of the plate and adjust the plastic wedge to permit this. Choose a stainless steel screw with a **thick** and **stiff plastic blank** to minimise the risk of the screw twisting during flask closure, (for heat-cured appliances).

- Wax up the bite to the height decided. Trim the wax bite-platform so that it has **just adequate antero-posterior depth.** If the bite-platform is too deep antero-posteriorly, then a significant percentage of patients will find it difficult to adapt from the point of view of speech and eating.

- **Heat cured acrylic is strongly recommended.** The acrylic dough is packed at a stage where it will flow well and not distort the position of the plastic blank holding the screw. The flask is closed slowly in a bench press.

- For appliances 6 iii & 6 iv the palatal springs should be kept **as flat to the tooth and palate as possible,** to minimise plaster boxing out and thicken the bite-plate. This reduces the risk of bite-plate acrylic fracture. Again use heat cured acrylic to maximise bite-plate strength.

ELSAA's with anterior bite-plates and NO anterior aligning wires
ELSAA's with anterior bite-plates and also anterior springs

FUNCTIONAL
APPLIANCE
DESIGN CARD

6

Functional Component Objectives

1. To expand the upper buccal segments 4-5mm.

2. To use this expansion to round out the upper labial segment (assisted by the incisal occlusion).

3. To use incisal function on the selectively rounded anterior bite-plate to tip instanding upper incisors and canines labially and to allow the lips to squeeze labially placed upper incisors and canines palatally as the overall arch perimeter is being increased.

4. To open the bite anteriorly with slight intrusion (and slight protrusion) of the upper and lower labial segments. There will also be a small element of backward hinging of the mandible which will need to be compensated for during the Class II displacement functional phase of treatment.

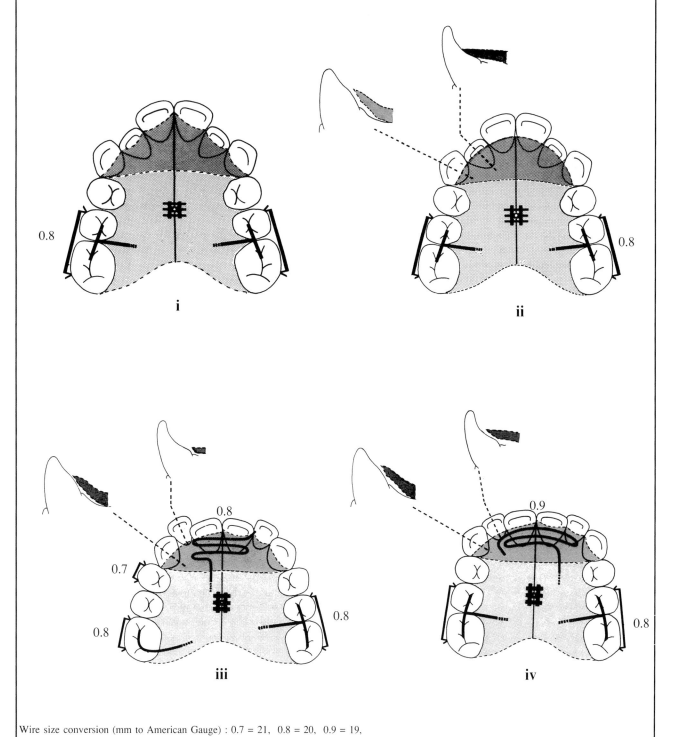

Wire size conversion (mm to American Gauge) : 0.7 = 21, 0.8 = 20, 0.9 = 19,

ELSAA's for MID - ARCH EXTRACTION cases, (4's or 5's)
ELSAA's for cases with EXTRACTION of UPPER 6's
or 6|6 Xbites

7

Clinical guidance on prescription

- Prescribe 7 i, 7 ii & 7 iii for any Class II Division 1 occlusions with profile retrognathia requiring a Class II displacement functional appliance, BUT in which the intra arch crowding is sufficiently severe to warrant mid-arch extractions of either 4's or 5's or 6's, as are clinically appropriate.

- In broad, general terms, **functional appliance cases work best** on a **non-extraction** basis or with **posterior relief of crowding** with loss of four second molars (4x7's), **if** the third molar position is satisfactory. **Significant crowding (more than 1/2 a premolar width) in a 32 unit dentition should always be relieved,** preferably at the back of the arches.

- **Substantial crowding (1 premolar width or more) is best relieved by extractions in the middle of the arches.** The choice between 1st and 2nd premolars is made on normal clinical grounds and is independent of the appliance design. Loss of first molars may be predicated by caries.

- Designs i, ii, & iii allow great flexibility in prescription and enable any variant of dento-alveolar crowding to be handled quickly and effectively.

- The aim is to produce an aligned arch, Class II Division 1 occlusion in which crowding has been relieved, which can then be sagittally corrected with a Class II displacement functional appliance; probably an activator variant eg Design Card 10.

- The clinician must stop thinking in conventional anchorage terms of the extraction site providing space for dental alignment; with this approach the **whole aligned maxillary arch** is providing anchorage for the Class II sagittal correction. Use design i for severe crowding and design ii for moderate crowding where loss of 4 x 5's is appropriate.

- The anterior spring in Designs ii & iii, together with the expansion, harnesses the often undervalued anchorage of 21|12 and induces worthwhile distal movement of premolars. This stout, but flexible, and certainly more versatile variant of the 'T' spring enables the correction of palatal Xbite on 6 at the same time as the upper arch is expanded. **The spring should NOT be covered with acrylic.**

- Design 7 iv is appropriate when differential buccal segment expansion is needed and when there is greater palatal positioning of 6's than the upper premolars.

- Lower mid-arch extractions can be handled well, initially with a buccal sectional arch, and later with full arch mechanics **within an activator treatment.**

Technical guidance on construction

- Crib choice and positioning need to be undertaken with care since they are an integral part of the appliance function and transmit the reciprocal of the palatal spring force to the premolars (Designs ii & iii).

- The technician needs to fully understand the clinician's intention for these subtle little appliances.

- As there is little acrylic the occlusal rests are critical to vertical support of the appliances and need to be placed with care.

- Palatal spring design should follow the advice given for Design Card 5 (technical guidance).

- The screws chosen should be **small** and fit well into the vault of the palate.

- The acrylic is an important functional component as well as being the linking medium. Anterior and posterior edge placing and finishing needs to be precise and to the clinician's, hopefully, well thought out design. Heat cured appliances are preferred.

- This group of appliances are amongst some of the most interesting and potent of the ELSAA's and should give the impression of being very neat and well made.

ELSAA's for MID - ARCH EXTRACTION cases, (4's or 5's)
ELSAA's for cases with EXTRACTION of UPPER 6's
or 6|6 Xbites

FUNCTIONAL
APPLIANCE **7**
DESIGN   CARD

Functional Component Objectives

1. Arch alignment prior to functional therapy, but taking account of :
   a) Occlusions requiring mid-arch extractions for relief of crowding.
   b) Occlusions requiring differential expansion across the premolars and molars (7 iv).
2. The harnessing of anterior anchorage to move premolars distally (7 ii & 7 iii).

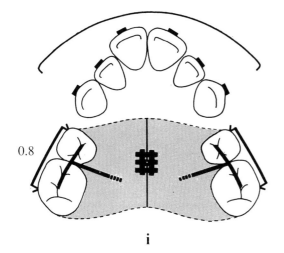

i

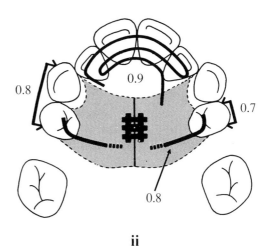

ii

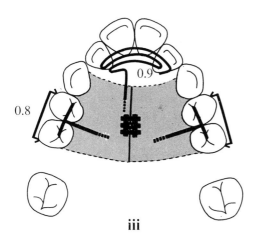

iii

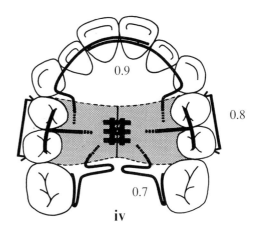

iv

Wire size conversion (mm to American Gauge) : 0.7 = 21, 0.8 = 20, 0.9 = 19

CHAPTER THREE

ACTIVATORS
DESIGN CARDS 8A -11

Activators may be defined as Class II displacement appliances having the major part of their functional components on the palato-lingual. The many activator designs that are described, are all descendants of the Andresen and are modifications designed to make the appliance **more tolerable**, eg the skeletal activators, the bionator, Kingston designs etc or to make the appliance **more effective** by means of headgear support, wire components, or greater bite opening eg the Van Beek, the Teuscher or the Harvold activators. One of the problems of name labelling of appliances is that clinicians may prescribe a name rather than undertaking a component analysis of the case to see which assembly of functional appliance components is most appropriate to the problem. This is the reason that the activators used at Kingston are described for their components rather than being named. There are two main variants of the activator design that have evolved at Kingston.

The Medium Opening Activator - Palatal (retained on the maxillary buccal segment)
DESIGN CARDS 8A, 8B, 9.

The Medium Opening Activator - Labial (retained on the maxillary labial segment)
DESIGN CARDS 10, 11.

These appliances work very well for the mild to moderate Class II Division 1 malocclusions having overjets of 8-10 mm with treatment taking about one year. For overjets well in excess of 12 mm it may take up to two years of favourable cooperation and response followed by a short course of fixed appliance therapy for final occlusal detailing. Additional care should be exercised in treating patients with an average to deep intermaxillary space, since an anterior open bite can develop due to over-eruption of the second permanent molars. In these situations an occlusal stop or acrylic block should be incorporated to control the mandibular second molars. Alternatively, an occlusal plane acrylic shelf as described by Harvold or as shown on Design Card 17 would be appropriate. If an anterior open-bite should develop (approximately 1 patient in 10) then it normally closes spontaneously over 6-12 months.

ACTIVATOR OR FRANKEL ?

A question which is frequently put during clinical assessment is whether an activator or Class II Frankel should be prescribed for a Class II Division 1 patient. The activator can be prescribed in similar circumstances to the Frankel and produces relatively similar skeletal and dental results but with small differences. The activators described are simple, robust, readily tolerated, less expensive, readily constructed, and work well for a broad spectrum of clinicians. The Frankel can work elegantly for some cases and on a visual examination appears to have a slightly better effect on lip form and function (this has not proved to be measurable). Frankel appliances are significantly less well tolerated on average than activators. Both appliance systems can be usefully used; but considerable experience of both is needed for the subtle deployment of the advantages of each. All appliances which cap the lower labial segment induce less proclination $(1-2^{o})$ of the lower incisors than a conventional FR (Design Card 1) which on average gives 5° proclination of the lower incisors with a range of -2 to $+14^{o}$. Lower incisor functional appliance capping is also better at bite opening in deep-bite cases. Activators induce more vertical descent of the lower border of the mandible than the conventional Class II FR.

ACTIVATORS - PALATAL OR LABIAL?

The Medium Opening Activator (MOA) - **Palatal** (Design Card 8A) **is designed for intact maxillary arch cases without buccal segment spacing.** It is our most commonly prescribed functional appliance which is reactivated at approximately 4-5 months as shown on Design Card 8B. If anterior brackets were used during the ELSAA phase of labial alignment, then Design Card 9 would be appropriate. The Medium Opening Activator (MOA) - **Labial** (Design Card 10) is used in cases **where there is spacing in the upper buccal segments** either naturally or as a consequence of extractions. The design permits natural space closure during the Class II labial segment correction. The cribbing is less secure than in the full palate activator and the spoon palate or the incorporation of 4|4 into the canine cribbing is intended to minimise rocking. The MOA - Labial design is useful, but only needed in approximately 1 in 5 of the activator cases. The appliance can also be used around anterior fixed appliances if these were used in the ELSAA phase (Design Card 11). If fixed appliances are needed **it is always better to consolidate the first premolar into the labial segment.**

THE PRE-ACTIVATOR PHASE OF ARCH ALIGNMENT

Cribbed activators on average are better tolerated and work better than loose activators (eg a conventional Andreson). For cribbed activators, a preliminary phase of arch expansion and alignment using the ELSAA appliance is needed in 19 cases out of 20. Provided this is planned and managed well it does not unduly extend treatment. The combination of ELSAA and Kingston activator designs means that the greater part of substantial Class II occlusion, Division 1 or 2, crowded or uncrowded, mid-arch or posterior arch extractions, can be handled with this system. High FMPA Class II Division 1 cases are best managed with the appliances described on Design Cards 14, 15, 16 or 17 as appropriate, subsequent to the initial maxillary arch alignment.

DENTAL ALIGNMENT

The skilful design of ELSAA and activator should permit maximised dental alignment by 'driftodontics' or 'nudgodontics'. There is frequently little need for a detailing of the occlusion using fixed appliances. Should this be necessary, full or sectional fixed appliances can easily be used in the lower arch **during** the activator phase of treatment. In difficult Class II cases with excess lower arch spacing to close (eg congenital absence of 5|5), the MOA provides valuable lingual support to the lower labial segment anchorage and eliminates its lingual tipping. This means that a moderate to severe Class II Division 2 case with moderate to severe upper and lower labial segment crowding can be converted into a Class II Division 1 case (non-extraction in the upper) and handled with mid-arch or lower labial segment extractions in the lower arch. Where sagittal arch correction has been fully achieved but the occlusion looks untidy **then** go into a full lower bond up initially, later followed by a full upper bond up. The lower bond up can be completed WHILST the activator is still being worn. Rapid nickel titanium arch changes allow the patient to be **into lower rectangular wires** BEFORE DISCARDING THE ACTIVATOR. With the upper arch full bond up (and therefore the cessation of the Class II displacement activator) there is thus a secure lower arch from which to use Class II elastic traction or a 'Jasper Jumper' to maintain the sagittally corrected arch relationship whilst final detailing of the occlusion takes place.

PATIENT INSTRUCTIONS FOR THE WEAR OF THIS RANGE OF MODIFIED ACTIVATORS Design Cards 8A, 9, 10, & 11

These are similar to the patient instructions for the wear of Frankel appliances but with a somewhat different emphasis due to the differences in design.

The appliance is a daytime as well as a nightime appliance. Over a 2-3 month period the patient should build up to 18-20 hours of activator wear. Concentrate on the daytime component during the first 2-3 weeks of wear. Provided the hole at the front of the activator is made as large as is technically feasible, then the majority of determined children will find that these activators do not significantly muffle speech. The lingually less dextrous child is frequently less cooperative and needs to be identified and remotivated by the 2nd or 3rd visit. By the second visit, satisfactory speech with the activator in the mouth is a measure of a treatment which will most probably go well. Since the appliance is clasped to the upper teeth the problems are different to the 'bounced Frankel appliance' but the solutions are the same. There are two rules:

1. The patient MUST **learn to speak with the teeth held together** with the lower labial segment firmly held into the lower labial capping. This is not easy for some children and is the reason why the first activator bite should be underactive (Design Card 8A). Children should read to their parents each evening during the first month of activator wear.

2. The appliance MUST, whenever it is removed from the mouth **be placed into its box** for security.

For the first 4-6 months of activator wear the fused ELSAA appliance (which should be kept in the same box) should be replaced in the mouth whenever the activator is removed to maintain the upper arch alignment. The activator will need to be removed, for meals and for some key lessons at school.

RETENTION OF THE SAGITTAL ARCH CORRECTION

At the end of the Class II displacement functional appliance phase of treatment (activators & Frankels) the patient should have arrived at a Class I incisal relationship with reduced overbite and overjet. This is referred to as a **Sagittal Treatment Complete (STC)** position and it should be recorded with a lateral skull film. The recently obtained STC position is at this point **unstable** and 1/3 to 1/2 of the overjet reduction **will be lost** if Class II displacement mechanics are immediately discarded. Frequently the sagittal correction is more rapid than the vertical adjustment of the buccal segments. The patient usually continues in the same functional appliance with the same wearing regime for 4-6 months whilst the buccal occlusion consolidates. With 10-20% of patients premolar eruption is very slow and more time will be needed. Where the buccal occlusion is very slow to settle, consider making an upper Hawley retainer, but with a wire which drops down from the anterior palate into position behind the lower labial segment to maintain the sagittal correction. This wire is similar in design to the lingual guidance wire used in the early Frankel designs. This type of retainer is however **only effective for patients who can adapt to keeping their teeth in occlusion most of the time.**

Where NO fixed appliance is needed.

No fixed appliances are needed for detailing the occlusion in 1 out of 2 Class II patients. In this case continue fulltime with the activator or Frankel initially but moving cautiously into a progressive withdrawal of the appliance. The patient can be seen three times a year and initially the appliance can be left out for mornings only, but otherwise it should continue to be worn afternoons, evenings and **at nights.** The choice of time of day does not matter but the advice wants to be positive, occlusally monitored and recorded, so that the clinician and patient can link cause and effect. Provided that the STC position is being substantially maintained, over approximately one year plus, move the patient to wearing the appliance **at night only.** At this point the patient will be into or approaching their pubertal growth spurt with still some facial growth to go. The patients will generally be grateful for the facial and occlusal improvement that has been obtained, particularly when shown the starting records, and will have sufficient self-interest to avoid any relapse. The mechanisms of further facial growth need to be explained and the patient asked to continue to wear the activator or Frankel at night only, until they know that their linear height is no longer increasing. The patient need only be seen twice a year for chat and encouragment and to put the appliance **through the ultra sonic cleaner.** Whilst this may seem a protracted treatment or maintainance regime, in reality it takes little clinical time, requires only an adequate recall system and gives quality facial and occlusal results to caring patients and parents.

A number of less motivated Class II displacement functional appliance patients who have lost their appliances, temporarily disappeared from the clinic etc, have shown that 1 in 4 of functional cases is very stable 6-9 months after arriving at the STC position. Since these cases are difficult to identify, long term retention is advised for all.

Where a fixed appliance IS needed.

Where fixed appliances are going to be needed for occlusal detailing it is important that a clear decision is made about this by one year into treatment. Patients will readily accept a declining functional appliance phase of treatment; **they will not readily accept a late decision to enter full fixed therapy.** Patients who are going to require fixed appliances (1 in 2 of functional cases) are more likely to have been treated with an ELSAA + an activator rather than a Frankel. Bonded edgewise brackets can easily be used in the lower arch during both the ELSAA and the activator phases of treatment. Where an activator induced STC position needs to be maintained during fixed appliance maxillary arch alignment then light maintaining Class II elastics or a Jasper Jumper (recent and relatively untried) is required. This needs a stabilised well aligned lower arch with a thick section rectangular wire in place. Nickel titanium wires are used nearly exclusively. The full fixed appliance phase of treatment should be completed in 6-9 months. Sagittal arch stability should be reasonably apparent by that stage. If in doubt add light headgear (usually through blob stops on a 0.8mm labial bow) to the maxillary retainer.

In summary, profile handicapping malocclusion can be treated in the mixed or early permanent dentition if possible without, but if necessary with, the use of fixed appliances. A nocturnal maintenance regime of the sagittally corrected arches should be continued until the end of the patient's growth in height.

TIMING OF TREATMENT START

Activators require a growing face, a tolerant patient and a dentition which is stable enough to support the system. **The minimisation of the risk of mixed dentition permanent incisor trauma is of major concern** in patients with medium to large overjets. If a robust, possibly accident prone child of average FMPA is seen in the early mixed dentition, then a Class II displacement functional appliance is prescribed. Treatment is NOT considered in the full **deciduous dentition** since most children up to the age of six would not tolerate the range of clinical procedures that are needed. Generally complete permanent upper incisor eruption and apical formation are required before the ELSAA phase of treatment can be initiated. Treatment starts can be considered throughout the mixed dentition until serious shedding of deciduous molars commences. At this point the rapid changeover of buccal segment teeth **may** make it difficult to get reasonable retention stability for the ELSAA or subsequent activator. A treatment start delay of 6-9 months, whilst the early permanent buccal dentition becomes established, may be appropriate with or without the active removal of loosening deciduous molars.

For choice, Class II Division 1 activator solvable problems are best treated in the early mixed or **mid-mixed dentition;** Class II Division 2 problems are best left until the **very early** permanent dentition to minimise the problems of protracted retention.

However many patients have been successfully treated with activators in the early years of the permanent dentition. Activators are more successful in the full permanent dentition than the Frankel appliances. **The further into the permanent dentition, then the more determined the patient will need to be to get a good result with an activator.** Determined patients of both sexes with moderate rather than very severe problems have been successfully treated into the mid-teens. In general however **permanent dentition treatments are more successful in the very early years** of the full permanent dentition.

FURTHER READING and REFERENCES - See Chapter Six

Technicians please note that in this chapter 'Technical guidance on construction' for Design Cards 8A, 10 & 11 is overleaf from the page 'Clinical guidance on prescription'.

Clinical guidance on prescription

- **Prescribe for Class II profile, low to average FMPA, mild, moderate, or severe Class II Division 1 occlusions, with average or increased overbites, and reasonably aligned lower and upper labial segments.**

- **Do not prescribe for very incomplete, reduced overbite or anterior open bite cases.**

- Initial upper labial segment crowding should be treated with an ELSAA appliance (chapter two).

- **Mild lower labial segment crowding** can be handled within the capping, by light alignment plastering and loss of 4x7's if appropriate.

- **Moderate to severe lower labial segment crowding** will require mid-arch lower premolar extractions and initially buccal sectional and possibly full arch lower fixed mechanics **to initiate alignment during the ELSAA phase of treatment.** Minimise the use of brackets on the lower incisors or place them more gingivally to avoid interfering with the acrylic capping. **Sectional retraction** of lower canines frequently results in **substantial spontaneous alignment** of lower incisors.

- If the patient has an average to above average maxillo-mandibular planes angle, **prescribe with caution.** Too much vertical development of $\overline{7|7}$ can prop the bite open and induce an anterior open bite. If the anterior, previously increased overbite reduces too fast or too extensively, then remake the MOA-palatal with a posterior occlusal acrylic block in the second molar region. If an anterior open bite is induced it will settle during the retention phase or fixed appliance phase of treatment.

- **The bite technique.** Identical to the Frankel on Design Card 1.

- **The bite objectives.** A slightly more active bite can be taken for the average activator patient as compared with a Class II Frankel (Design Cards 1 & 2) ie 4-6mm forward and 2.5-3.5mm open buccally. Use the lower end of the range for the small and timid patient (see Design Card 8B for reactivation).

- **Impressions.** Standard good impressions are needed, particularly on the lingual of the lower labial segment. A thin roll of white beading wax should be placed in this area. If the edge of the lower tray perforates the impression on the lingual of $\overline{4|4}$ then the working impression should be retaken.

See overleaf for technical guidance on construction

Functional Component Objectives

1. Sagittal restraint of forward growth of the maxilla & maxillary dentition.
2. Vertical restraint of maxilla & maxillary dentition.
3. Total freedom for eruption of lower buccal segments.
4. Vertical restraint of the lower labial segment.
5. Maximised increments of the condylar growth mechanism. (Gives an added increase of mandibular corpus length by approximately 1-1.5mm per annum during the period of active appliance wear).
6. Forward & vertical mandibular guidance along the Y-axis giving an enhanced mandibular dentition movement relative to the maxillary dentition, and the induction of a Class I buccal occlusion.
7. Increase in the ratio of lower to total face height.
8. Minimised uprighting of the upper incisors (average 10°).
9. Minimised proclination of the lower incisors (average $1-2^{o}$).
10. To translate a Class II Division 1 incisor relationship into a Class I relationship with a reduced overjet and overbite.

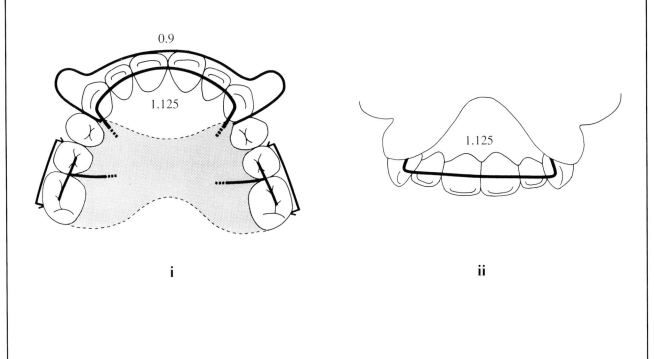

i   ii

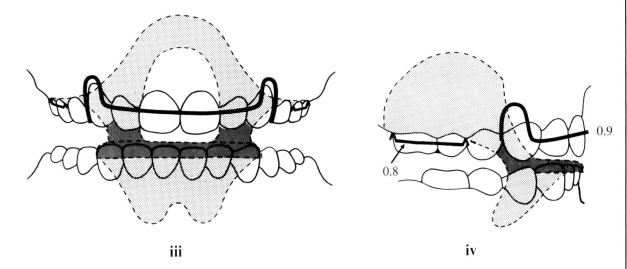

iii   iv

Wire size conversion (mm to American Gauge) : 0.8 = 20, 0.9 = 19, 1.125 = 17

Technical guidance on construction

- Rinse and dry the impressions and cast them in a mixture of 50% stone and 50% plaster.

- Since good access will be needed from the BACK of the working models, use a casting technique which minimises the need for trimming on the lingual of the lower model.

- It is critical to remove the lower impression without fracturing the lower incisors. If this happens, don't bodge it - recast, and take more care next time.

- Trim the lower and upper model so that there will be good vision from the **back** of the models once they are articulated. Do not cut into the lingual mucosa impression area behind the lower incisors since this area is critical for an accurate atraumatic fit of the lower labial capping.

- See that the working models seat into the bite and articulate on a plane line or plasterless articulator with the anterior teeth pointing towards the articulator pillar. This later allows maximum access from the back in the final waxing stage of linking the capping to the upper.

- **Remove** the articulator and **only then** take off the bite. If a plane articulator is opened on its hinge with the bite in place there is a strong chance of fracturing the lower incisors.

- At this point check the bite. Look at the models held in maximum intercuspation (ie the patient's normal bite) and see that the active bite is within the limits outlined in the clinical guidance on 'bite objectives'. If the bite is too open, too forward or lopsided or the centrelines are significantly off, then contact the clinician before proceeding.

- Examine the lower labial segment alignment. If there is any degree of $\overline{3211123}$ crowding think how this may be allowed to spontaneously align **within** the capping. Undertake minimal finger plastering on the lingual of labially displaced incisors. The capping must be in contact with the tips and **lingual surfaces of most of the lower labial segment teeth.**

- **A common technical fault** with this appliance is to **overplaster the lower labial segment** and produce a baggy fit of the capping. The patient doesn't quite know where to close and is able to move the mandible within the capping. This can result in soreness or stripping of the mucosa on the lingual of the lower incisors.

- Complete the maxillary wirework. Wire sizes (in mm) are:

Labial bow	0.9 ideal in form with 1-1.5mm of buccal relief of 3l3. The horizontal part of the wire is placed as high gingivally as the interdental papillae permit, and the bow has medium sized 'U' loops.
Palatal wire	1.125 as ideal in form as possible and well up on the cingulum of 21l12 towards the incisal tip, to minimise uprighting of the upper incisors. The palatal wire must also be rested on the cingulum of 3l3 . **Do not overwork** the wire in this area since it is a common fracture point. Use 1.0mm wire for a small arch.
Buccal cribs	0.8, a double crib on 65l56 or 6El E6 is favoured. Reduce the wire size to 0.7mm if cribbing premolars.
Occlusal rests	These 'butterfly' occlusal rests are made from a 1.0mm cross type clasp fabricated by Krupps for wrought denture clasps.

- Complete the upper wax work on the palatal of 654l456, wax to above the survey line.

- Lower incisal capping. Wet the lower model, and **closely adapt** one sheet of non brittle wax, eg Tenatex. Trim the outline required. Lay a second sheet over the first, then smooth, outline, and seal to the first sheet.

- Lift off the capping, check the smooth, but well-contoured inner surface, rearticulate and check that the bite is not gagged on the lower capping.

- To form the pillars two small pieces of well softened wax are placed, sealed in and shaped to link the upper working model to the lower capping.

- This capping, which is now attached to the upper waxed appliance, is lifted off the lower model and invested in plaster in a deep activator flask in a similar way to an Andresen appliance.

- Note. **THE AUTHOR PREFERS A HEAT CURED APPLIANCE FOR STRENGTH AND EASE OF REACTIVATION.** Technicians who prefer to make the appliance in autopolymerising resin should link the lower capping to the upper with 1.5mm wire.

Functional Component Objectives

1. Sagittal restraint of forward growth of the maxilla & maxillary dentition.
2. Vertical restraint of maxilla & maxillary dentition.
3. Total freedom for eruption of lower buccal segments.
4. Vertical restraint of the lower labial segment.
5. Maximised increments of the condylar growth mechanism. (Gives an added increase of mandibular corpus length by approximately 1-1.5mm per annum during the period of active appliance wear).
6. Forward & vertical mandibular guidance along the Y-axis giving an enhanced mandibular dentition movement relative to the maxillary dentition, and the induction of a Class I buccal occlusion.
7. Increase in the ratio of lower to total face height.
8. Minimised uprighting of the upper incisors (average 10°).
9. Minimised proclination of the lower incisors (average $1-2^o$).
10. To translate a Class II Division 1 incisor relationship into a Class I relationship with a reduced overjet and overbite.

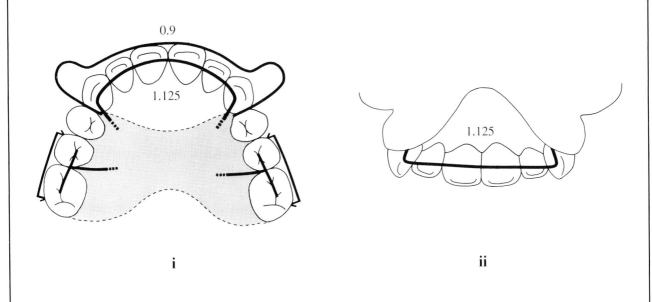

i   ii

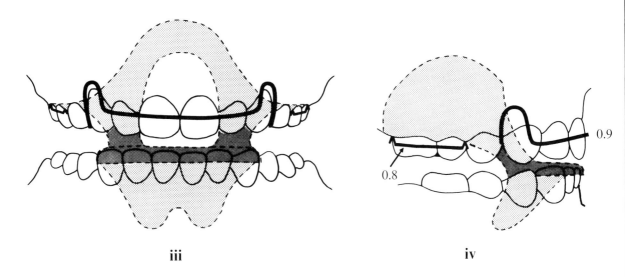

iii   **iv**

Wire size conversion (mm to American Gauge) : 0.8 = 20, 0.9 = 19, 1.125 = 17

Clinical guidance on reactivation

● With functional appliances, **patient tolerance is all.** The clinician should have taken an initial bite which would be tolerated by the patient (albeit with some effort and encouragement). If there had been any concern by the clinician about tolerance then **an underactive bite should have been taken.**

● At the first check visit (4 weeks) investigate every aspect of patient compliance, reassure and re-encourage.

● At the second check visit (4 weeks) the patient should be starting to settle well (and with growing confidence) into the appliance. If so dismiss for 6-8 weeks.

● **If not, then a serious patient and parental discussion is appropriate** with a further 4 weekly review to ensure that compliance is now fully forthcoming. If by the fourth visit cooperation is still not at an acceptable level, then a major review of treatment objectives is appropriate with parent and patient. It may be necessary to give up the attempt at a worthwhile functional appliance-induced profile improvement, consider changing the type of functional appliance, consider extracting four premolars and using fixed appliances, consider a Herbst appliance (Design Card 18) or even an orthognathic approach. NO FUNCTIONAL APPLIANCE CASE SHOULD DRIFT PAST FOUR MONTHS WITHOUT REAL PROGRESS BEING SEEN TO BE MADE.

● By 3-4 months the bite will only be active by 1-2mm; at this point, the activator should be advanced.

● Using a fine straight fissure bur, section the acrylic pillars along the section line shown in the diagram.

● Using a large tungsten carbide acrylic trimmer, shorten the pillars but leave the base so that the technician can reshape the new pillar from this point.

● Holding the lower capping on the lower labial segment, **practice the patient** in the reactivated bite position.

● Take a sheet of non-brittle wax, roll it into a well softened ball about 1.5 centimetres in diameter and then squash this down into the anterior palate leaving a small surplus roll of softened wax hanging down from the upper incisal tips.

● Again place the capping onto the lower incisors, get the patient to **gently** close into the **previously practiced** bite, **stay** and **hold.**

● The clinician should check the centrelines, the advance and the degree of buccal bite opening. Make sure that the patient **stays** in the desired bite.

● The chairside assistant should then pass a warmed (but not excessively hot) wax knife and with the patient's lips well retracted, the clinician should lightly seal the wax onto the acrylic lower labial segment capping.

● Gently remove the now advanced Medium Opening Activator, check that the sealing of the capping is adequate, lay it on a soft padding of wet tissues in a protective box and pass it to the laboratory for reconstruction of the acrylic pillars.

● Expect this to be completed on a **same day turn around, am to pm,** so that there is no loss of continuity of progress.

● At the pm refit warn the patient that it will feel different and that they may need to rework their way into the appliance. Check that the lingual of $\overline{21|12}$ doesn't develop any soreness; if so, relieve.

● **This reactivation regime is appropriate to Design Cards 8A, 9, 10 & 11.**

Technical guidance on reactivation

● On receipt of the advanced activator, a plaster bed needs to be made, which will record the bite taken and ensure that the capping does not move while the acrylic struts are being reconnected.

● Lay a small bed of plaster on the bench, **gently** add some plaster into the capping and then embed the appliance, labial bow down, into a bed of plaster. One side of the bed should support the palate of the appliance, the other side of the bed should support the capping.

● When the plaster has set, boil out the wax, and roughen the area to be acrylated with a bur.

● Now add pieces of wax to shape the form of the acrylic pillars and produce the anterior breathing hole. This is a 'fiddly business', but time spent pays dividends in finishing later. At this point one can see the value of the clinician leaving the base of the original pillar (clinicians please note).

● Activate the roughened area of acrylic well with monomer before adding the autopolymerising acrylic and then pressure cure.

● The new acrylic polymerised struts are a potential weak link. The material used must be of a good quality and handled well. The strut will also be mechanically at risk because it will be angled forward at a more acute angle. Some small increase in the length of the 'oval' of the strut cross-section may be appropriate. Bear in mind the fact that the breathing hole wants to be kept as large as possible.

● Provided this advice is followed the advanced Medium Opening Activator rarely fails at the strut.

● Complete the fine shaping of the acrylic struts with tungsten carbide trimmers and polish well.

● If the advance is undertaken whilst the patient waits, allow over one and a half hours of laboratory time. This will allow for waiting time whilst plaster and acrylic set.

Functional Component Objectives

INITIAL BITE TAKING:

A 4-6mm initial sagittal **advance** is appropriate for most patients with a range of 3-8mm. The more the bite is **opened** in excess of 2.5mm the less the sagittal advance should be.

Most patients initially develop a long centric slide from their habitual to their most retruded condylar position. The length of this slide usually reduces progressively over a short time period.

REACTIVATION:

As soon as the activator is only active by 1-2mm (normally at 3-5 months) it should be advanced and reactivated. The advance should be approximately 3mm with a 1-2mm further vertical opening.

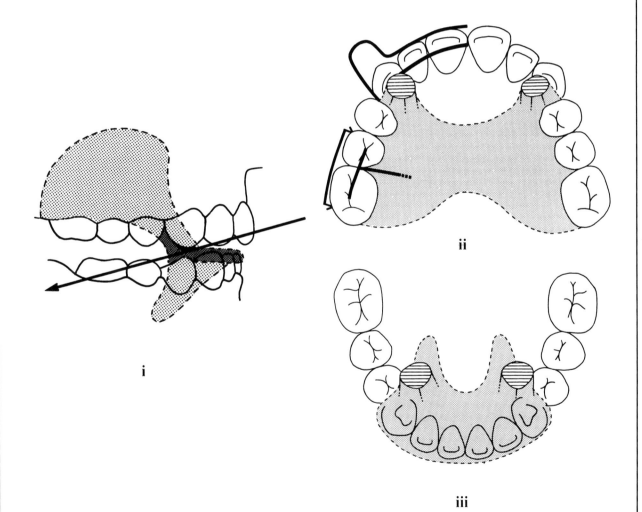

i

ii

iii

Clinical guidance on prescription

- **Prescribe for Class II profile, low to average FMPA, mild, moderate, or severe Class II Division 1 occlusions, with average or increased overbites and a reasonably aligned LOWER labial segment (similar to Design Card 8) BUT WITH A PREVIOUSLY VERY IRREGULAR UPPER LABIAL SEGMENT** (this will have been aligned using Design 4 iii or 4 iv).

- If anterior brackets are inevitable to align 3＋3 in addition to the ELSAA appliance, then it is usually better to bond back to 4|4 as in 9 ii and use a single crib on 6|6 only. The consolidated labial segment including the first premolar gives a better labial anchorage unit if there should be some posterior upper buccal segment spacing and the need to consider Design 11 ii.

- The presenting occlusion may initially have had set back 2|2 in which the clinical crowns were shortish with some gingival hyperplasia on the mesio-labial. This rarely resolves until the brackets are removed and patients with indifferent oral hygiene may easily acquire white decalcification scars on the labial of 2|2 . This should be watched carefully and **if in doubt remove the brackets** and cope with the tendancy to reimbricate by other means, eg an ELSAA as in Design 7 iii.

- **All patients with any fixed appliance or removable appliance with buccal overlays should be on daily fluoride mouthrinses.**

- The initial (now fused screw) ELSAA appliance should be worn whenever the activator is out of the mouth (meals, sports and verbal lessons at school).

- If the initial occlusion had a very imbricated upper and **lower** labial segment a clinical decision will be needed on whether mid-arch relief of crowding is required in **both arches** (Design 7 i & ii followed by a variant of Design 10 i & ii or Design 11 i & ii) or whether loss of $\overline{4|4}$ can be combined with 7|7 extraction. Whilst leaving an atypical buccal occlusion, extraction of $\frac{7|7}{4|4}$ can work out very well in some cases of this type.

- If extraction of $\overline{4|4}$ is appropriate, start lower sectional mechanics of the type described by Orton & McDonald in the E. J. Orthod. 7: 120-126, 1985 at the start of the upper arch ELSAA phase of treatment.

- As a consequence of lower canine retraction, the lower incisors will frequently spontaneously align enough for the lower capping to function well without bonding the lower incisors. If $\overline{21|12}$ need to be actively aligned bond the brackets slightly low (watch the oral hygiene) and align the incisors prior to fitting the activator.

- **Do not start intra-traction for space closure** UNTIL the activator is worn well. The activator will stabilise the lower labial segment well forward and avoid the risk of uprighting and retroclining the lower incisors in a Skeletal II case.

- Since fixed appliances need to be worn for the shortest time possible (and always less than a year if feasible), do delay the entry into fixed appliances as much as is realistic during the ELSAA and activator phase of treatment. It is easier to design and support these appliance systems in the absence of brackets. Once basic arch alignment and sagittal arch correction are completed with appliances that are removable from the mouth, it is relatively easy and quick (6-9 months) to detail the occlusion with upper and lower fixed appliances.

Technical guidance on construction

- The advice given for the construction of the Medium Opening Activator-Palatal (Design Card 8A) should be followed in detail since this is an almost identical appliance.

- When the upper working model has been cast, the plaster cast of the brackets may need some small amount of neatening up, since the alginate impression material easily tears in this area.

- The labial wire, size 0.9mm, should be tightly in contact with the brackets and incisal to them.

- The labial wire has no 'U' loops for adjustment and is contoured neatly around the distal of the last tooth in the bonded segment ie 9 i around 3|3 or 9 ii around 4|4 .

- The length of the labial bow will affect the pattern of cribbing.

- Otherwise technical guidance for Design Card 9 is identical to that for Design Card 8A.

Functional Component Objectives

1-10. Similar to Design Card 8A.

11. Maintains the incisal alignment following the use of an ELSAA with anterior brackets. (This style of appliance is only used when the starting upper labial segment imbrication is marked).

NOTE : The modified labial bow lies incisal to the brackets and the arch wire does not incorporate 'U' loops. This design of arch holds the anterior teeth together and its position, incisal to the brackets, aids in bite-opening (view iii).

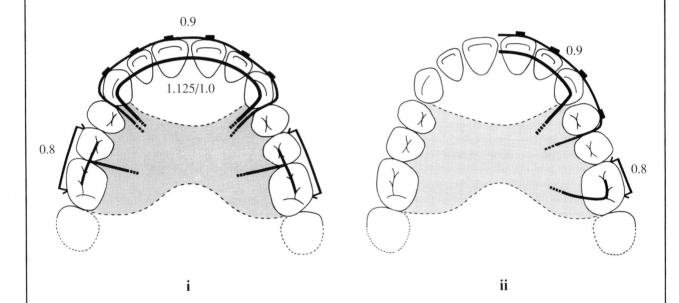

i

ii

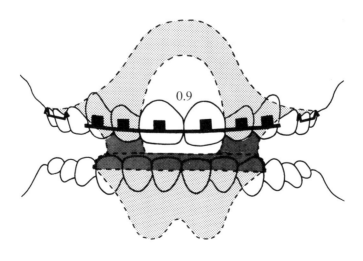

iii

Wire size conversion (mm to American Gauge) : 0.8 = 20, 0.9 = 19, 1.0 = 18, 1.125 = 17

Clinical guidance on prescription

- **Prescribe for Class II profile, low to average FMPA, mild to moderate Class II Division 1 occlusions with average or increased overbites and UPPER BUCCAL SEGMENT SPACING.**

- The degree of the upper buccal segment spacing may well have been determined by the consolidation of labial segment spacing previously present or induced during the ELSAA phase of treatment.

- Any SIGNIFICANT anterior open spacing should always be consolidated prior to the activator phase of treatment, from 3 + 3 or **preferably** 4 + 4.

- MARGINAL anterior spacing should be gathered up during the final fixed appliance phase of treatment.

- The MOA-Labial is clinically a less potent appliance than the MOA-Palatal due to problems of retention and rocking.

- Consolidation of spacing from 4 + 4 rather than 3 + 3 minimises these problems.

- It is not an appropriate activator for **severe** skeletal II cases. Where this type of case has upper arch spacing the anterior spacing should be consolidated from 4 + 4 and an MOA-Palatal used which will hold the space consolidated distal to 4|4. This first activator, plus one advance, will deal with the worst of the retrognathia. When this is mild to moderate **then** prescribe the MOA-Labial, to consolidate the upper labial segment to the upper buccal segment.

- Final detailing of this type of clinical problem usually requires upper and lower fixed appliances supported by Class II traction.

- The entry into **lower** fixed appliances should be undertaken **during the last four months of activator therapy,** so that a rectangular arch wire can be in place in the lower to support the Class II traction to the upper arch when the activator is discarded.

- MOA-Labial design features. Wire sizes (in mm) are:

Crib 3|3	0.7 upper canine cribs give good retention but check that the palatal acrylic is well up on the cingulum. If not, canine extrusion may be induced. Six months plus of canine cribbing may induce canine tipping, particularly if the labial bow is slack.
Crib 43|34 + occlusal rest	0.8 double cribs give excellent retention with little rocking, particularly if a 0.8mm rest is laid into the occlusal fissure of 4 from the mesial. This wire is not shown on Fig 10 ii to avoid making the diagram too complex.
Labial bow	0.9 from 3 + 3, use slightly squared 'U' loops which just clear the 3|3 cribs. **Never** solder the bow to the bridge of the cribs. If double cribs are used on 43|34, then use even squarer 'U' loops with the wire passing **underneath** the bridge of the double crib to enter the acrylic distal to 3|3.
Acrylic	The acrylic spoon palate should cover the maximum area to minimise rocking, consistent with posterior edge tolerance and clearing the buccal segment teeth for mesial drifting and eruption. THIS ACTIVATOR MUST BE MADE IN HEAT CURED ACRYLIC.

NOTE This useful activator has a limited place and is prescribed for approximately 1 in 5 of activator solvable problems. This group will include ELECTIVE MID-ARCH EXTRACTION CASES (see Design Card 7). The MOA-Labial can be advanced by the same techniques as in Design Card 8A.

See overleaf for technical guidance on construction

Functional Component Objectives

1. General activator indications (Design Card 8A, functional component objectives 1 & 3-10) BUT **use in the presence of upper buccal segment spacing.**
2. Vertical & labio-palatal restraint of the upper labial segment only.
3. Vertical restraint of the lower labial segment.
4. Total freedom for eruption & mesial migration of teeth in the upper and lower buccal segments.

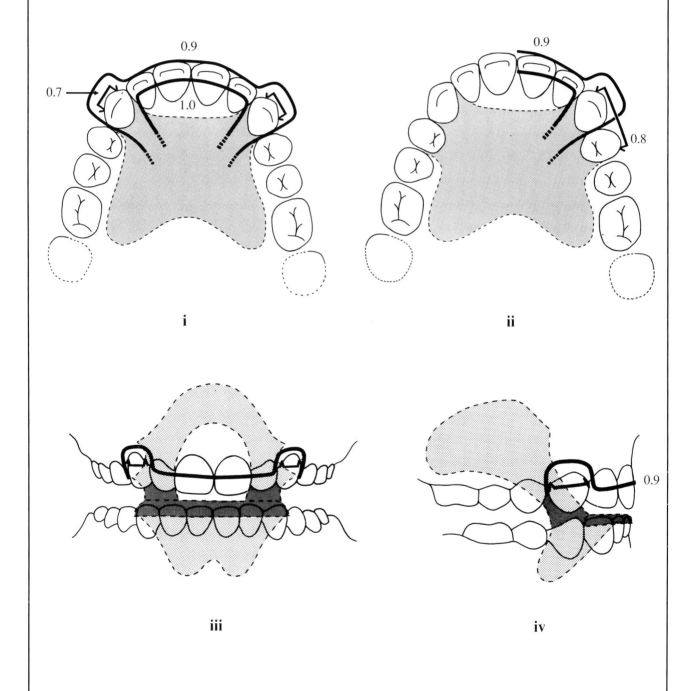

i

ii

iii

iv

Wire size conversion (mm to American Gauge) : 0.7 = 21, 0.8 = 20, 0.9 = 19, 1.0 = 18

Technical guidance on construction

- The impression handling, articulation, lower labial segment plastering and lower labial segment capping techniques are identical to those already described for the MOA-Palatal (Design Card 8A).
- The main construction variation is in the maxillary wire and acrylic work. Wire sizes (in mm) are:

3I3 cribs	0.7. The bridge of the cribs should not be too long and the arrowheads want to be more vertical than with a molar crib, with the tip of the arrowhead right at the gingival margin of 3I3 .
Labial bow 3 + 3	0.9. 3I3 **cribs should be made first and lightly tacked into position.** The labial bow from 3 + 3 should have the incisal portion as high as the interdental papillae will permit, and with squarish, but not too large or flexible, 'U' loops to sweep round the 3I3 cribs. The wire enters the acrylic on top of the distal leg of 3I3 cribs.
Labial bow 3 + 3 but in the presence of double cribs on 43I34	0.9. When double cribs are prescribed the **labial bow** should be **bent first.** The distal legs of the 'U' loops should be closely contoured to the buccal interdental embrasure, since the bridge of the double cribs will pass buccal to these wires.
43I34 double cribs	0.8. These very effective cribs should have their bridge cranked to follow the natural curve of the premolar and canine but stay buccal to the labial bow. Keep the mesial arrowhead slightly more vertical than the distal arrowhead.
Occlusal rests on 4I4	0.8. A further aid to minimising appliance rocking is to place occlusal rests into the fissures of 4I4 . The foot of the labial bow needs to be kept slightly to the mesial to allow these wires to enter the occlusal fissures of 4I4 . Note that these wires **are not drawn** on Fig ii to avoid making the drawing confusing. The occlusal rests on 4I4 are only prescribed when double cribs are used on 43I34 .
Palatal wire 21I12	1.0. This wire should be ideal in form and well up on the cingulae of 21I12 . The wire wants to be as heavy as possible since it is prone to fracture.
Wire entry palatal to 3I3	This is a very busy area for wirework; the feet of the cribs, palatal wire and labial bow, should neatly run into the acrylic on a parallel (not crossed) course with at least 1.0mm of space between each wire.
Maxillary wax-up	**The appliance can only be made satisfactorily in heat cured acrylic.** The palatal of 3I3 is a key area and the wax wants to be well up on the cingulae of the canines to prevent canine extrusion. The outline of the spoon palate will depend on whether a single or double crib is used. The lateral edge of the spoon should clear the premolars and molars by approximately 2mm. The posterior edge should be a smooth recessed curve from the disto-palatal of the first molars.
Acrylic struts wax-up	This is a little more awkward than for the MOA-Palatal. The anterior breathing (and speech) hole needs to be as large as possible consistent with satisfactory strut strength.
Acrylic finish	In view of the relative delicacy of this complex but effective little appliance, use a high quality, strong, heat cured acrylic. Enlarge the breathing hole if appropriate and polish well. Finish the edge of the spoon palate to a tapered but slightly rounded margin. It should be finished about 3mm from the palatal aspect of the posterior teeth.

Functional Component Objectives

1. General activator indications (Design Card 8A, functional component objectives 1 & 3-10) BUT **use in the presence of upper buccal segment spacing.**
2. Vertical & labio-palatal restraint of the upper labial segment only.
3. Vertical restraint of the lower labial segment.
4. Total freedom for eruption & mesial migration of teeth in the upper and lower buccal segments.

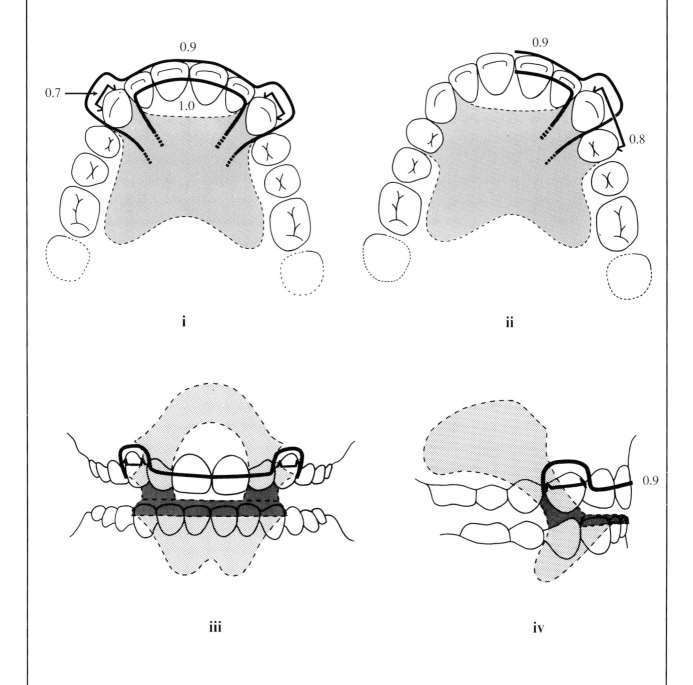

i

ii

iii

iv

Wire size conversion (mm to American Gauge) : 0.7 = 21, 0.8 = 20, 0.9 = 19, 1.0 = 18

Clinical guidance on prescription

- **Prescribe for Class II profile, low to average FMPA, mild to moderate Class II Division 1 occlusions with average or increased overbites AND GENERALISED UPPER ARCH SPACING, or previously severe upper incisor rotations.**

- The upper anterior spacing should be gathered together using a combination of anterior brackets (3+3, or **preferably** 4+4) and an ELSAA (Design 4 iii or iv).

- The general clinical guidance is similar to Design Card 10 for management and prescription, and Design Card 8A for the bite.

- **A good upper working impression is needed** which should show the bracket outlines well. It is important to **remove the upper archwire** prior to taking the impression. The same archwire should be replaced and 3+3 or 4+4 linked with secure but passive ties. It is important that **there is no anterior tooth movement between the working impressions and fitting the appliance.**

- Teeth which have brackets on them will have been moved mesio-distally and may also have been derotated. These will be unstable unless well ligated onto a stable, passive archwire.

- In all functional appliances where there is a risk of tooth movement between the impressions and fit, there wants to be the quickest possible turnround of appliances between impressions and fit, eg one week if possible. However, ALL FUNCTIONAL APPLIANCES SHOULD BE MADE WITHIN A TWO WEEK TURNROUND BETWEEN IMPRESSIONS AND FITTING THE APPLIANCE. (**This cannot be emphasised too strongly**).

- Where clinicians, technicians, nursing or reception staff tolerate a four week or four week plus appliance turnround then the patient failure rate of settling into the appliance rises sharply. It can be a very expensive delay.

- The appliance drawings (Figs i & ii), show the flexible retention clips in 'exploded view'. These clips lie against the labial surface of 32|23 and engage the gingival undercut of the brackets on these teeth.

- In all activator cases treated with an ELSAA appliance, the lateral buccal segment expansion is very unstable at the start of activator treatment and should be controlled by wear of the ELSAA whenever the activator is out of the mouth.

- Lower and then upper full fixed appliances will most probably be needed to finish the case, with a similar approach to that outlined for Design Card 10.

See overleaf for technical guidance on construction

Functional Component Objectives

1. General activator indications (Design Card 8A, functional component objectives 1 & 3-10). Also use in the presence of upper buccal segment spacing.

2. There are however a number of clinical situations (eg spaced upper arch Class II Div 1 problems), where it is clinically appropriate to seek Class II mandibular forward displacement as well as having the ability **to close anterior spacing either during the ELSAA phase or activator phase of treatment.**

3. A Medium Opening Activator-Labial can incorporate a localised fixed appliance from 3+3 or from 4+4 .

4. This type of problem invariably finishes up in upper and lower fixed appliances to complete the detailing of the occlusion.

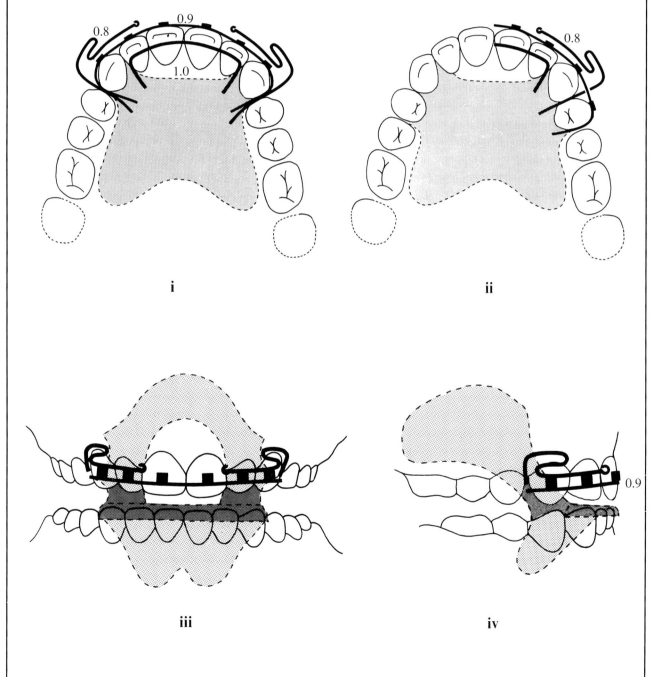

i

ii

iii

iv

Wire size conversion (mm to American Gauge) : 0.8 = 20, 0.9 = 19, 1.0 = 18

Technical guidance on construction

- The impression handling, articulation, lower labial segment plastering and lower labial segment capping techniques are identical to those already described for the MOA-Palatal (Design Card 8A).

- The palatal wire, maxillary wax-work and acrylic finishing are identical to those already described for the MOA-Labial (Design Card 10).

- The labial bow in 0.9mm wire lies incisal to the brackets and is identical to the bow already described for the MOA-Palatal with anterior brackets (Design Card 9).

- It is hoped at this point that the technician will appreciate **the assembly of similar technical components** to produce appliances that **will cope with moderately differing dento-alveolar circumstances** in faces that do however **have an underlying similarity of skeletal problem.** Effectively **a functional component analysis has been undertaken.**

- The only item that is unique to the MOA-Labial with anterior brackets is the 0.8mm flexible wire clips. The retentive portion of the wire lies **gingival** to the brackets on 3|3 or more commonly on 32|23 .

- It will be seen from the description of the labial bow and the flexible wire clips that an accurate impression of the labial segment brackets is a necessity. This is the reason that the maxillary impression technique has been stressed in the clinical guidance for this appliance.

- On receipt of the maxillary impression in the laboratory the impression should be rinsed and **gently** dried. Any partially torn alginate around the brackets should be eased back into place - if feasible - before casting.

- On removal of the alginate, undertake any light plaster trimming around the brackets that seems appropriate.

- MOA-Labial with anterior brackets design features. Wire sizes (in mm) are:
  The palatal wire, acrylic outline and lower incisor capping are identical to Design Card 10.

The labial bow	0.9. This wire lies just incisal to the brackets and enters the acrylic distal to the bonded canine or preferably the bonded first premolar, if this tooth has been included in the anterior sectional mechanics. The wire gives a firm intrusive component and sagittal restraint of the upper labial segment. This promotes the closure of the upper buccal segment spacing.
The retainer clips	0.8. The appliance is retained with these flexible clips which lie gingival to the brackets on 3|3 or more commonly on 32|23 . Exploded views (Figs i & ii) are shown to avoid confusion.

- A new functional appliance is difficult for any child to accept and tolerate. **A new functional appliance which is a poor fit is readily rejected by most children.**

- There must therefore be as short a period as possible between the impressions and the fitting of all functional appliances.

- **Design Cards 9 & 11** should be returned to the clinician for fitting **by one week from the impression date if possible** and certainly by no more than two weeks.

- IN GENERAL **ALL** FUNCTIONAL APPLIANCES (activators, Frankels and intrusive appliances) SHOULD BE MADE AND FINISHED IN THE LABORATORY SO THAT THERE IS NO MORE THAN TWO WEEKS BETWEEN THE IMPRESSIONS AND THE FIT OF THE APPLIANCE.

Functional Component Objectives

1. General activator indications (Design Card 8A, functional component objectives 1 & 3-10). Also use in the presence of upper buccal segment spacing.

2. There are however a number of clinical situations (eg spaced upper arch Class II Div 1 problems), where it is clinically appropriate to seek Class II mandibular forward displacement as well as having the ability **to close anterior spacing either during the ELSAA phase or activator phase of treatment.**

3. A Medium Opening Activator-Labial can incorporate a localised fixed appliance from 3+3 or from 4+4.

4. This type of problem invariably finishes up in upper and lower fixed appliances to complete the detailing of the occlusion.

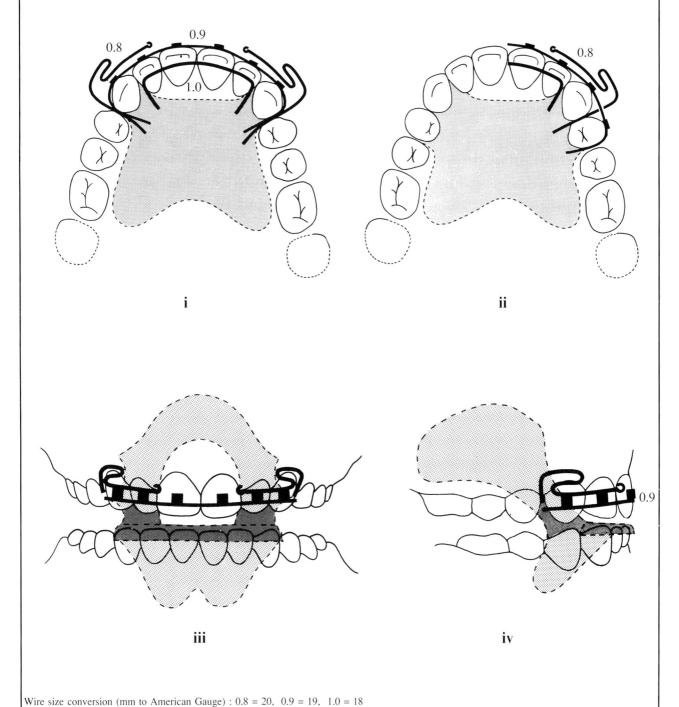

i

ii

iii

iv

Wire size conversion (mm to American Gauge) : 0.8 = 20, 0.9 = 19, 1.0 = 18

PREFABRICATION OF AN 'INTRUSIVE' HEADGEAR BLANK
USED FOR APPLIANCE DESIGN CARDS 14-17
(Completion of the fabrication is illustrated on Design Card 12A.)

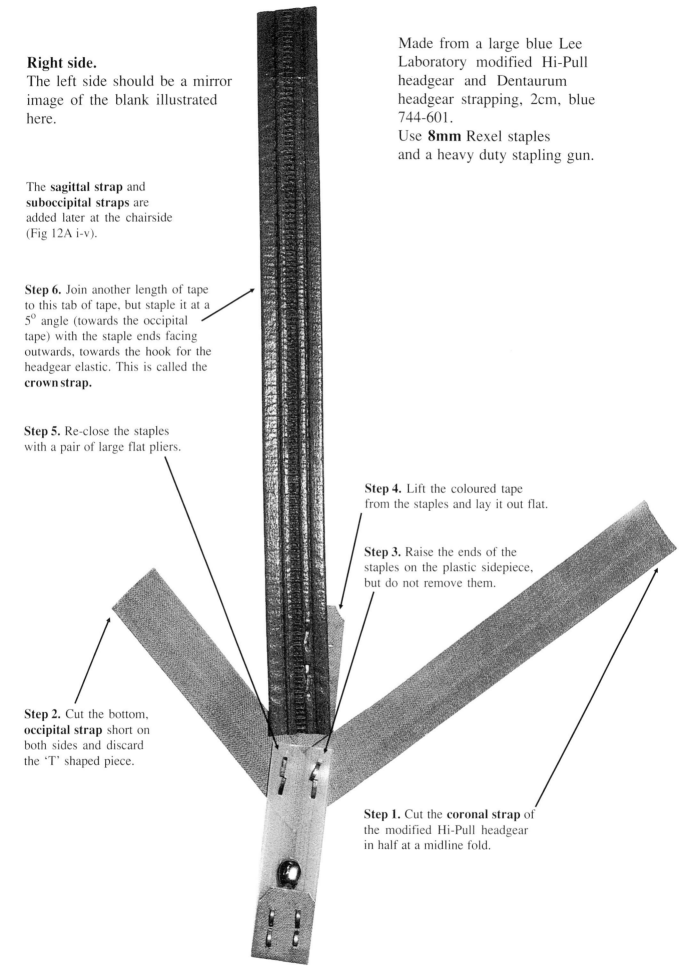

Right side.
The left side should be a mirror image of the blank illustrated here.

The **sagittal strap** and **suboccipital straps** are added later at the chairside (Fig 12A i-v).

Step 6. Join another length of tape to this tab of tape, but staple it at a 5° angle (towards the occipital tape) with the staple ends facing outwards, towards the hook for the headgear elastic. This is called the **crown strap.**

Step 5. Re-close the staples with a pair of large flat pliers.

Step 2. Cut the bottom, **occipital strap** short on both sides and discard the 'T' shaped piece.

Made from a large blue Lee Laboratory modified Hi-Pull headgear and Dentaurum headgear strapping, 2cm, blue 744-601.
Use **8mm** Rexel staples and a heavy duty stapling gun.

Step 4. Lift the coloured tape from the staples and lay it out flat.

Step 3. Raise the ends of the staples on the plastic sidepiece, but do not remove them.

Step 1. Cut the **coronal strap** of the modified Hi-Pull headgear in half at a midline fold.

CHAPTER FOUR

'INTRUSIVE' FUNCTIONAL APPLIANCES
DESIGN CARDS 12-17

All Class II displacement functional appliances (eg activator variants and Frankels), increase the lower anterior face height. This is now well recognised and contraindicates the prescription of activators and Frankels in:

- High FMPA cases.

- Cases with a wedge shaped intermaxillary height, either by virtue of an increased lower anterior face height or alternatively, by virtue of a very reduced posterior face height with a normal anterior lower face height.

- Cases with an overall long face.

- Patients with a gummy smile, usually Class II Division 1, but sometimes Class II Division 2.

- Bimaxillary protrusion skeletal II cases in combination with marked lip inadequacy with the lips at rest failing to cover the gap between nose and chin by 5-15+mm.

- Cases with anterior open bite (AOB).

In all of these groups the clinician seeks some control of the vertical descent of the upper buccal and labial segments. This vertical control may need to be undertaken:

- Usually **evenly** on the buccal and labial segments together (Design Cards 15, 16 & 17).
- Sometimes **differentially with more upper buccal** than upper labial intrusion, eg anterior open bite cases (see Design Cards 13 iii-vi, & 14).
- More rarely **with more labial intrusion** than buccal intrusion, eg gummy Class II Division 2 malocclusion (see Designs 5 i & ii).

Treating these malocclusions with fixed appliances can give difficulty, in that all fixed appliances tend to slightly extrude buccal segment teeth particularly when combined with Class II traction. Intrusive headgears applied to fixed appliances are of limited effectiveness. Slight extrusion of posterior molars in a wedge-shaped intermaxillary space may produce a significant worsening of any tendency towards anterior open bite. Unless the clinician develops techniques for the vertical control of the maxillary dentition, he is substantially handicapped in his management of the long faced Class II Division 1 problem.

A truly intrusive headgear is difficult, if not impossible, to fabricate due to the anatomy of the skull. The further forward the headgear attachment is taken (ie the more vertical the pull) the greater the tendency for the headgear to fall forwards off the forehead. A judicious modification of a simple Hi-Pull (modified Lee Laboratory) headgear has allowed the headgear hook to be taken forwards from just in front of the ear to just behind the outer canthus of the eye. A very stiff whisker and its stiff insertion into a rigid acrylic plate allows the transmission of mainly intrusive and minimally retrusive forces to the upper buccal segments by means of buccal overlays and to the upper labial segment by means of incisal capping. This approach to treatment can only take place during a period of growth. A recent treatment versus control group study showed that during the period of treatment, approximately 2 mm of suppression of vertical development of the maxillary dentition could be expected. The intrusive effect of the headgear is augmented by the buccal overlays and the occlusion.

This group of appliances divides into a number of systems:

THE BUCCAL INTRUSION SPLINT (BIS) - Design Card 14

This appliance is used to treat skeletal anterior open bites (AOB) by intrusion of the upper buccal segment teeth. This allows an element of forward mandibular hinging with a 4-6 mm spontaneous reduction in overjet as well as closure of the anterior open bite.

THE MAXILLARY INTRUSION SPLINT (MIS) - Design Card 15

This appliance is used to treat Class II Division 1 patients with a gummy smile. The upper incisors intrude approximately 2+ mm relative to the resting length of the upper lip and upright by approximately 10°. This uprighting should be minimised by using the deepest possible incisal capping and by a soccer goalpost shaped wire on $\underline{\text{III}}$. The overjet will reduce by 6-7 mm. Forward mandibular hinging can occur but is less predictable than one would wish. There is frequently unwanted excess eruption of lower buccal segment teeth to compensate for the suppression of eruption of the upper molars. This lower buccal eruption can be further controlled with an intrusive activator (Design Card 17). The MIS is most appropriate for small overjet (6-8 mm), gummy, Class II Division 1 occlusions. Some upper arch expansion and rounding out is best undertaken with an ELSAA **prior** to the MIS.

THE MIS PLUS A LOWER TRACTION PLATE - Design Card 16

The probability of forward mandibular hinging can be increased to a small, but useful extent, by using elastic traction from a 'concorde' design extra-oral traction whisker to a lower traction plate. This technique has been adapted, with acknowledgments, from Bill Clark's Twin Block technique. It can be used successfully in 8-14mm overjet cases. The forward mandibular displacement is less predictable than with the intrusive activator. The system is more easily tolerated than the intrusive activator.

THE INTRUSIVE ACTIVATOR - Design Card 17

The most effective appliance currently employed for the treatment of severe long faced Class II Division 1 malocclusion is the intrusive activator. This appliance gives a very positive maxillary vertical control and the buccal inter-occlusal acrylic minimises unwanted lower buccal segment eruption. A positive forward mandibular displacement is ensured by the lower acrylic and a relatively rapid maxillary and mandibular response is seen. The appliance **muffles** speech and is a 14/24 hours rather than an 18-20/24 hours appliance. To make a difficult appliance tolerable the lingual acrylic must have minimal thickness and the bite must not be too active. The appliance cannot be reactivated and up to three remakes may be needed to treat a severe problem. Whilst this may be expensive, the appliance system is a very satisfactory way of handling a very difficult malocclusion and brings into an orthodontic treatment range, long faced Class II Division 1 malocclusions with overjets of 10-18mm. This concept has evolved from a combination of the MIS and Van Beek's headgear modification of the Harvold appliance. We do not, however, employ the very open bites of the Harvold technique since many patients (nearly 1 in 2) are unable to settle into this appliance system.

THE CLARK TWIN BLOCK

The principles of this system have been most valuable in the development of a comprehensive functional appliance components concept. Whilst the appliance has been tested, it is not described here since most Class II malocclusion is already covered by the other appliances described in Design Card 8A for low to average FMPA Class II Division 1's, and Design Card 17 for high FMPA severe Class II Division 1's. The principles of the buccal bite blocks forward mandibular displacement and in particular the differential control of wedge-shaped buccal open bites are shown visually in Design Card 13, so that the reader may appreciate the important basic principles which can be applied when there is the need to 'personalise' a functional appliance for a particular patient (Ref : *E. J. Orthod.* 4: 129-138, 1982). Any clinician seeking to become a fluent prescriber of functional appliances should be very familiar with this article. The appliance system is particularly appropriate for moderate Class II Division 1 cases **with very incomplete overbites,** markedly wedge-shaped intermaxillary spaces and **WITHOUT** over-visible upper incisors during expressive behaviour.

INTRUSIVE   HEADGEAR   FABRICATION

There is no satisfactory, manufactured, intrusive headgear available giving comfort, with a traction position that provides maximum intrusion and minimal retrusion. In view of the variation in head size there is always likely to be the need to customise the headgear from patient to patient. A modified Lee Laboratory Hi-Pull headgear is used as the basis for adaptation, and the suboccipital and crown straps are made from a reinforced paper tape. This is then stapled using heavy duty 8mm staples. It takes time to aquire the skills to customise these headgears, but when experienced it should take the clinician 5-10 minutes to make a good headgear. The chairside time taken to prefabricate the headgear can be shortened by getting the orthodontic assistant to prefabricate headgear blanks as shown on page 52. It is always worthwhile making the headgear at the appliance impression visit, and placing it in a headgear bag containing elastics in a range of strengths (see Design Card 12A). The clinician can then concentrate on the more important matter of **patient motivation** at the appliance fit visit.

TIMING   OF   TREATMENT   START

The advice on timing of treatment start for intrusive appliances is similar to that given for activators on page 35. Patients, both young (8 years) and through to the early teens (13-14 years) will wear headgears well. Since 'intrusive mechanics' relies on the suppression of vertical facial growth, then there must be growth to come. Treatments progress well in the mixed-dentition. Permanent dentition treatments should be initiated as early as possible and preferably by the beginning of the pubertal growth spurt. The later the treatment start relative to the start of the pubertal growth spurt, the more determined the patient must be. Intrusive treatments do not succeed after the cessation of facial growth.

FURTHER   READING   and   REFERENCES   -   See Chapter Six

Technicians please note that in this chapter 'Technical guidance on construction' for Design Cards 14, 15, 16 & 17 is overleaf from the page 'Clinical guidance on prescription'.

Clinical guidance on fabrication

- Although a small number of attempts have been made there is no marketed, satisfactory, **intrusive** as opposed to high pull, headgear.

- There is a fundamental incompatability between the shape of the calvarium and the relative forward placement of the maxillary denture from the point of view of producing a headgear which gives intrusion only. It is not possible to produce a headgear force which gives intrusion without retrusion.

- A major purpose of the clinical routine outlined subsequently is to produce a headgear that **maximises the intrusive component** and **minimises the retrusive component.**

- Take a modified Lee Laboratory Hi-Pull Headgear. This has a hook portion, a coronal strap, and an occipital strap. The occipital strap has attached to it a sagittal strap that is normally loose but is custom fitted to the patient and then stapled to the coronal portion.

- Cut the coronal strap in the midline (page 52 step 1) and the occipital strap (page 52 step 2) so that there is 6cm of strap distal to each hook portion. On each hook portion in turn lift up the two staples and unfurl the folded-over piece of tape (page 52 steps 3 & 4). Bend the two staples back down again (page 52 step 5). The unfolded piece of tape now projects between the coronal and occipital portion. To it is attached 20cm of headgear paper tape (known later as the crown strap) angled slightly backwards towards the occipital strap (page 52 step 6). The portion can be prefabricated by the dental surgery assistant. A photograph of an intrusive headgear blank for the right side is shown on page 52 for the guidance of the dental surgery assistant. The left side should be a mirror image of this.

- The patient then holds the hook portions of the headgear firmly on the face immediately distal to the outer canthus of the eye (page 59, Fig 12B i). The coronal straps are folded over each other in the midline to form a shallow V, slightly forward of the anterior fontanelle. These straps are marked and stapled (Fig 12A i).

- The patient again holds the hook portions in the same place. 40cm of tape (the suboccipital tape) is then held over the base of the occipital arm of the prefabricated portion. It is marked and stapled **on one side only** (Fig 12A ii). The headgear is replaced and the suboccipital tape is gently tightened, marked and cut to the required length and stapled on the other side (Fig 12A iii). The headgear will already start to fit. Spare tag ends of the occipital arm of the prefabricated portion can be cut off.

- The midline of the suboccipital strap is marked and a 30cm tape added to pass along the line of the sagittal suture (Fig 12A iv). This is then taken **under** the point of the shallow V of the coronal strap and gently tightened back on itself before being marked and stapled.

- We now have a vertical headgear which fits snugly and has two unstapled ends of tape (the crown straps) projecting towards the crown of the head (as shown in Fig 12A iii). It is these two tapes that will, when secured, take the main weight of the intrusive appliance on the crown of the head.

- The patient now holds the headgear hooks gently downwards and forwards, whilst the crown straps are led under the sagittal strap and gently tightened to feel the pull of the patient's fingers. The crown straps form a natural V. The position of the straps is marked, slightly tightened to make more weight, stapled to each other and the sagittal strap, then any spare end tags are removed (Fig 12A v).

- Whilst this may seem a complex procedure, it takes less than 10 minutes when the clinician is familiar with it. It is however a procedure **that should be out of the way** when the patient is being inducted into the management of their intrusive appliance. **The headgear should be made when the design, bite and impressions are undertaken.**

- The headgear should be issued to the patient in a headgear bag with **a graded series of elastics** that will give from 75 to 400+ grams of pressure. If these packets of elastics are numbered with a routine numbering system, both clinician and patient know where they are. The patient is expected to progress to 400 grams of pressure bilaterally in 2-3 months. The very light starting force of 75 grams is not biologically very effective but is merely to get the patient **used to the system.**

- **See page 58,** Design Card 12B 'Fabrication of the linking system to intrusive appliances' **for the legends appropriate to photographs 12A vi, vii & viii.**

The fabrication of THE VERY HIGH PULL 'INTRUSIVE' HEADGEAR

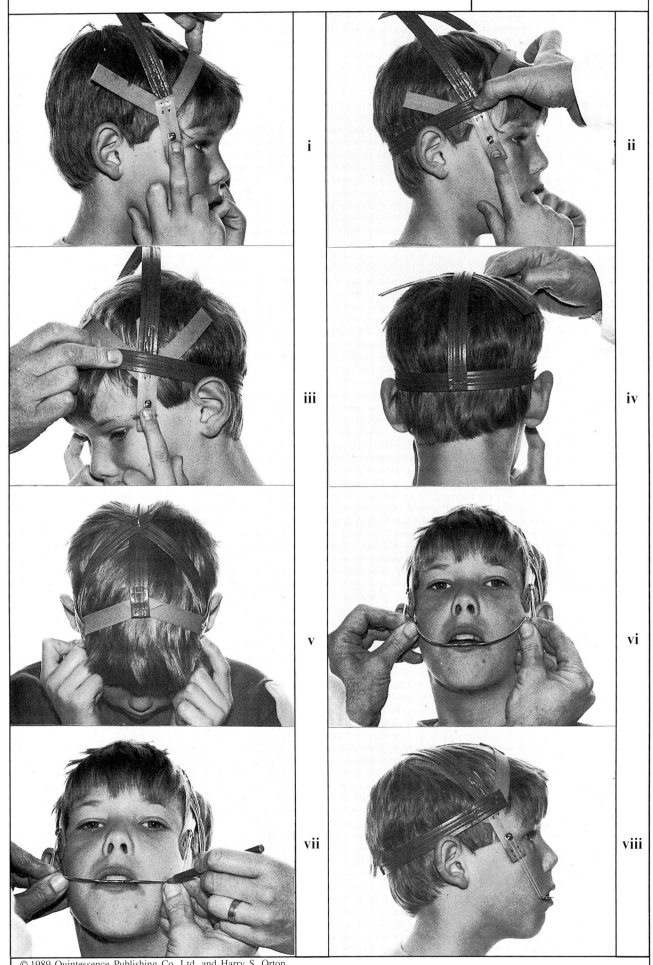

i

ii

iii

iv

v

vi

vii

viii

Clinical guidance on fabrication

- The extra-oral facebow is inserted into a large internal dimension headgear tube (.051") which has an absolutely rigid insertion into the acrylic of the appliance. The mesial of the tube is usually at the tip of the cusp of 4|4 and this gives **a short and rigid internal bow** which can only be removed from the tubes with difficulty. This minimises the risk of inadvertent ocular damage.

- The stiff external bow should be shaped to the face and should be a piece of 1.8mm wire which is relatively unyielding over the 5-6cm of wire that will be needed when the outer whisker has been adjusted for length..

- **The hook of the headgear should be partially closed** so that a heavy elastic will only just 'ping' into it (for ease of headgear handling and safety).

- The patient should be **sat upright in the dental chair**, with the intrusive appliance in and the headgear positioned with a pair of heavy (300 gram pressure) elastics in the hooks. The clinician should sit comfortably in front of the patient with the patient's head turned slightly towards the clinician.

- The clinician should **hold the elastic tightly between the tips of the forefinger and thumb** and run his **thumb-nail** backwards and forwards along the outer whisker, feeling the **pull of the elastic** and the **flex of the outer bow.**

- When the thumb-nail is towards the back of the outer bow (Fig ii) the bow will tip up at the back and the appliance will feel as though it is coming down at the front (see page 57 Fig 12A vi).

- When the thumb-nail is towards the front of the outer bow (Fig iii) it will feel as if the appliance is being intruded on the incisors and the back of the appliance is coming down.

- There is a certain position on the outer bow between these two states, and specific to a millimetre, where it feels as if ALL the maxillary teeth included in the appliance are being intruded (Fig iv and see page 57 Fig 12A viii).

- Feel this position once or twice and then get the dental surgery assistant to mark the thumb-nail position with a sharpened, wax marking pencil (see page 57 Fig 12A vii).

- Cut the wire 6mm distal to the mark and smooth the end of the wire. At this point ANNEAL the end of the wire from the end to 2mm past the mark. Apart from being difficult to bend, unannealed wires may fracture and ruin the precision of the whole exercise.

- Take the end of the wire in the base of a pair of strong spring forming pliers and slowly but smoothly roll in a hook. Nearly close the hook with a pair of large flat grooved pliers so that the elastic 'pings' into the hook (for security of the system).

- The hook on the outer bow is further forward, with a shorter external whisker than many clinicians would expect on a theoretical consideration of the system (see page 57 Fig 12A viii).

- If the intrusion is **directed at the buccal segments** only (Design Card 14), rather than the whole maxillary arch, THEN **the external whisker will be longer.**

NOTE The security of the system from the point of view of ocular risk is excellent. The rigid internal bow is extremely stiff and is only removed with physical difficulty from the headgear tubes. If the bow is experimentally pulled out, the mechanics of the system, impacts the bow under the external nares. A 'Mazel' plastic safety strap can be added routinely if required. If this is used it is important that it is sufficiently loose to avoid placing any distal force on the headgear bow. If the intra-oral functional appliance is ONLY used when the headgear and the Kloehn bow are in place, then the ends of the internal whisker can be made to protrude 2-3mm beyond the distal of the flying EOT tube. These protruding ends can be turned up (and slightly in) to permanently lock the bow into the tubes.

Functional Component Objectives

1. To have a stable, comfortable headgear, **with the traction hook as far forward as possible** in order to produce an intrusive force on the maxillary dentition. The limiting factor to forward positioning of the hook is the outer canthus of the eye (Fig 12B i).

2. To take account of the patient's calvarium shape, hair style etc, to produce a stable and comfortable intrusive headgear which the patient will tolerate well.

3. To produce an appliance and **linking system** which will deliver a safe intrusive force, to part or the whole of the maxillary dentition.

4. **To minimise the retrusive** component of force on the maxillary teeth **and maximise the intrusive** component.

5. This approach is used with :

   the Buccal Segment Intrusion Splint   Design Card 14
   the Maxillary Intrusion Splint   Design Card 15
   the Maxillary Intrusion Splint + Clark type lower   Design Card 16
   the Intrusive Activator   Design Card 17

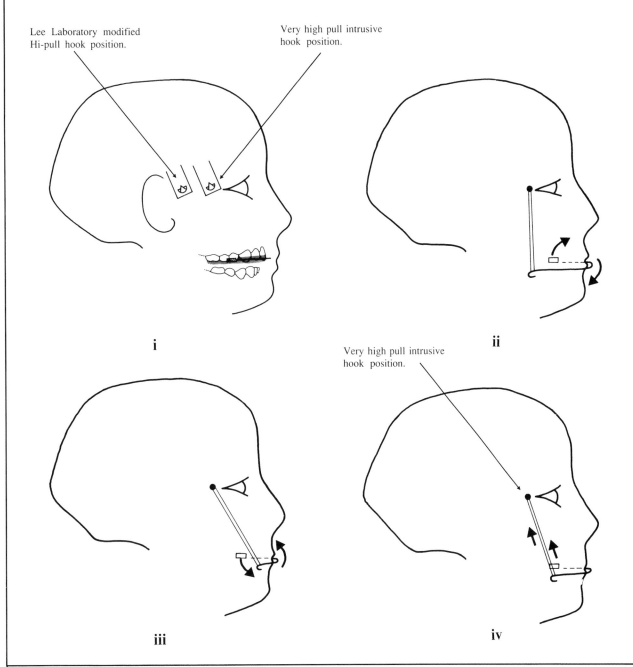

Lee Laboratory modified Hi-pull hook position.

Very high pull intrusive hook position.

i

ii

Very high pull intrusive hook position.

iii

iv

Clinical guidance on prescription

- The orthodontic and dental profession is indebted to Mr WJ Clark of Kirkcaldy, Scotland for the development of this innovative Clark Twin Block (CTB) system which has been a valuable functional contribution to functional appliance prescription.

- **The appliance system is particularly appropriate for moderate Class II Division 1 occlusions with very incomplete overbites, markedly wedge-shaped intermaxillary spaces and WITHOUT over-visible upper incisors during expressive behaviour.**

- Whilst the system has a number of strengths it does induce buccal open bites and **it is therefore less appropriate for DEEP-BITE Class II malocclusions which are better treated with modified activators.**

- This apparent short-coming of the system can however be taken advantage of, **to cause forward mandibular hinging with reduction of anterior open bites and small reductions in overjet (4-6mm).**

- Superimposition on anterior cranial base of tracings of treated cases shows the shadow of the mandibular symphysis travelling forwards by 1-2mm and slightly upwards by 0-1mm, rather than showing the downwards displacement that would normally be expected during a Class II displacement functional appliance treatment.

- Cases with AOB from $\frac{3+3}{3+3}$ and small overjets (4-8mm) are treated with the buccal intrusion splint (BIS, Design Card 14). In these cases Clark's lower anterior block is incorporated into the upper appliance and intrudes the lower rather than the upper premolars.

- Cases with anterior open bite extending further posteriorly ie from $\frac{4+4}{4+4}$ or from $\frac{5+5}{5+5}$ are initially treated with a shortened buccal wedge buccal intrusion splint eg fig vi. If the clinician wishes to use a CTB system in these circumstances then the lower anterior block is taken out of occlusion with $\underline{4|4}$ eg Fig iv.

- If the overjet is large and a more active forward traction is needed, then a Clark type lower traction plate, WITHOUT A BUCCAL BLOCK (Design Card 16 iii), is used with the traction hooked to a 'concorde' whisker (Design Card 16 i). This type of whisker can be employed with either a buccal intrusion splint (Design Card 14) or with a maxillary intrusion splint (Design Card 15).

- Once an anterior open bite has been closed with a buccal intrusion splint, review the patient's smile line, and if this still gives a 'gummy' appearance, then switch into a maxillary intrusion splint.

- If an element of anterior vertical maxillary incisal control is needed but still with a main element of posterior molar intrusion then the MIS (Design Card 15) can be waxed up with a posterior thickening of the buccal overlay occluding against the lower first molar, eg Fig vi.

- The combination of a MIS with a posterior Clark block and a standard lower Clark plate with a lower block has been tried but does not give any worthwhile clinical advantage.

- For cases which employ these principles, bites should be taken which are rather more open (3-4.5mm) than many functional appliance bites (2-3mm).

Functional Component Objectives

1. The Clark Twin Block has as its primary purpose the induction of a forward displacement of the mandible.

2. Secondarily the buccal blocks may induce intrusion of some or all of the buccal segment teeth depending how the blocks are constructed (Figures ii, iv & vi).

3. If an incomplete or anterior open bite is present then the buccal intrusion results in a slight forward hinging of the mandible with closure of anterior open bite.

4. The Clark buccal block concept is used (at Kingston) primarily as a technique to close anterior open bites.

5. The blocks may be designed as in :

Fig ii   to close an anterior open bite from $\frac{3+3}{3+3}$

Fig iv   to close an anterior open bite from $\frac{4+4}{4+4}$

Fig vi   in association with an elastic from the lingual of a lower removable appliance upwards and forwards to an anterior hook on a 'concorde' headgear whisker to close an anterior open bite from $\frac{5+5}{5+5}$

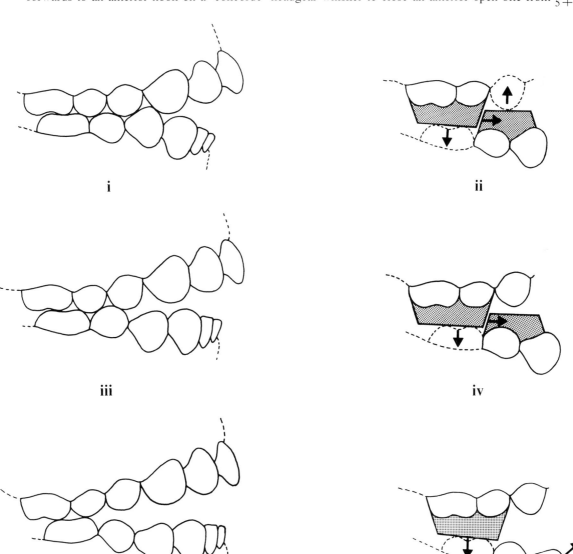

i

ii

iii

iv

v

vi

THE BUCCAL SEGMENT INTRUSION SPLINT (BIS)

Clinical guidance on prescription

- **Prescribe for Class II occlusions with anterior open bite or very incomplete overbites.**

- Cases with a localised $\frac{3+3}{3+3}$ region AOB of mild dimension, ie less than 3mm, **which is associated with obvious digit sucking** and an average to low FMPA, **should be left to await cessation of the habit.**

- Most AOB's of a significant dimension have a skeletal as well as a dento-alveolar component with increased lower anterior face height both in relation to the upper anterior face height and the lower posterior face height.

- The most important single component is the excessive vertical development of the upper buccal dento-alveolar segment. Intrusion of $\underline{6}$ relative to the maxillary plane, by approximately 2mm, is the objective of the appliance system.

- This amount of upper buccal segment intrusion will result in forward mandibular hinging with closure of the anterior open bite and a 4-6mm reduction in overjet.

- The consequence of the AOB closure is generally to leave a slightly reduced Class I overbite.

- **Appliance design.** First look at the extent of the anterior open bite which may be localised anteriorly, or may extend posteriorly to include the premolars or sometimes even the first molars.

- **Only the teeth in occlusion should be overlaid.**

- This will affect the cribbing pattern and may result in $\underline{64|46}$ single cribs, $\underline{65|56}$ double cribs, or $\underline{6|6}$ single cribs only.

- **The further back the AOB extends, the further distally the flying headgear tube should be placed.**

- A midline screw should be placed, but the stiff and short inner bow of the headgear whisker prevents it working in more than a minor way to compensate for distal movement of the buccal segments.

- **If substantial upper arch expansion is needed, then gain this expansion first,** with the BIS alone, expanding the screw 1/8 turn per day. If necessary replace the screw and **add in** the headgear at the end of 2-3 months.

- The palate is relieved by the technician so that the full intrusive occlusal and headgear pressure is taken on the teeth which are propping the occlusion (Fig iii).

- **Clinical preparation.** Write a 'thought-out appliance prescription', then take upper and lower standard working impressions and a bite. The bite should be in maximum intercuspation with enough anterior wax to support the AOB working models without them tipping. **The headgear should be prepared in advance when the working models are taken.**

- This allows the clinician to concentrate on fitting the linking system (Design Card 12B) and motivating the patient when the system is placed.

- **Patient Instructions.** The buccal overlay appliance should be worn full time including meals. The headgear and whisker is added for as many hours of the day and night as the patient can **reasonably** tolerate. This wants to be at least 12 in every 24 hours or ideally more.

- Unless active crossbite correction is sought (see above) activate the midline screw one 1/4 turn per week.

- If extraction of $\underline{7|7}$ is planned, **delay this** until AOB closure is completed. $\underline{7|7}$ may be forced buccally off the ridge, but their presence minimises distal movement and tipping of the upper buccal segments. It is of course important that **the buccal capping controls $\underline{7|7}$ vertically during this phase.** If extraction of $\overline{7|7}$ is planned, then undertake the lower extractions **prior to** the start of the BIS treatment to maximise spontaneous alignment in the lower arch.

See overleaf for technical guidance on construction

Functional Component Objectives

1. Maximised intrusion of the upper buccal segment teeth that are propping the occlusion. (Intrusion and supression of growth is about 2mm).

2. Minimised retrusion and distal tipping of the upper buccal segments. (If 7|7 extraction is planned it is better to leave 7|7 in situ until the intrusive phase is completed. But if $\frac{7|7}{7|7}$ extractions are planned continue with $\overline{7|7}$ extractions from the start of treatment).

3. Minimised eruption of the lower buccal segments. (Rebuild the upper buccal overlays 3-4 months into treatment).

4. Total freedom for spontaneous vertical development of the upper and lower labial segments.

5. Reduction in the anterior open bite by differential vertical development, or suppression, of the labial and buccal segments respectively.

6. Reduction of the anterior open bite by forward mandibular hinging giving spontaneous overjet reduction of 4-6mm. This consequence is only of value in the Class II case.

7. Reduction of the lower anterior face height as a percentage of total face height by 1-2%.

NOTE To conform with standard user convention (UK & USA) **the tubing sizes only** are shown in thousandths of an inch.

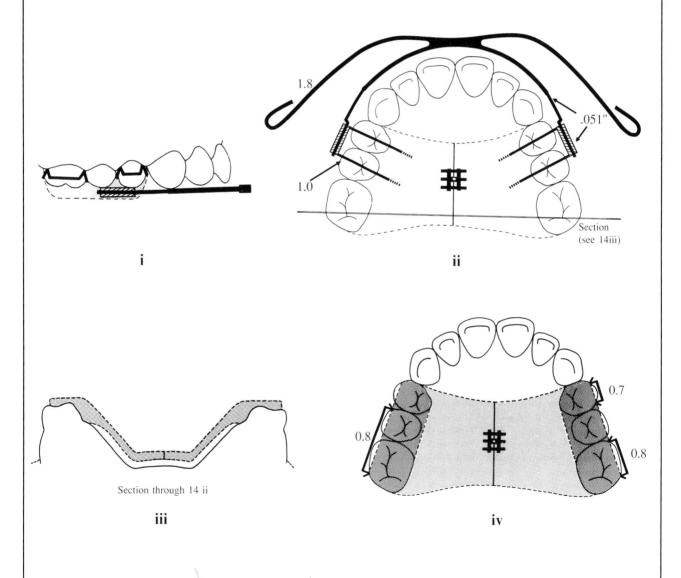

i

ii

Section
(see 14iii)

Section through 14 ii

iii

iv

Wire size conversion mm to American Gauge) : 0.7 = 21, 0.8 = 20, 1.0 = 18, 1.5 = 15, 1.8 = 13

Technical guidance on construction

- Rinse and dry the impressions and cast them in a mixture of 50% stone and 50% plaster.

- Take the upper model, note the area to be covered by the appliance and then WAX THE PALATE filling any indentations or rugae, to give a smooth waxed palate which extends 2mm forwards and backwards of the intended area of the BIS. **Do not wax into the gingival margins** of the upper buccal segment teeth (Fig iii).

- Then warm and lay a single sheet of non-brittle wax, eg Tenatex, and press this smoothly into place avoiding thinning the sheet in the middle of the palate. Shape and seal the sheet in place. The wax relief should be 1.5-2mm thick.

- **It is important** that the palatal gingival margins and palatal surfaces of 654|456 **are not waxed out** (Fig iii). The waxing should finish 1-1.5mm from the gingival margins of 654|456 **otherwise the cribs will not be retentive.**

- **Then duplicate** the working model and make the BIS on the duplicate model.

- Articulate the palatally relieved upper working model and the lower working model on a hinged articulator in the maximum intercuspation bite obtained by the clinician.

- Open the vertical dimension screw on the hinge so that a buccal overlay of adequate thickness can later be waxed up. A compromise is required between patient tolerance and adequate thickness to avoid any risk of breakage of the buccal blocks. Since **the blocks must not fracture during use,** these are generally 2mm thick at the tip of the cusp.

- The cribs are made and waxed in place with a little plaster laid on the wire running across the interdental embrasure. This stops the trans-embrasure part of the crib becoming embedded in the acrylic and losing its flexibility. **Interdental embrasure plastering must always be done when Adams's clasps are covered with a buccal overlay.**

- The flying headgear tube should be 6mm long and taped and soldered to a piece of 1.0mm wire that has been previously bent into a squared-off 'U'. 0.051" tubing is used to give a stiff inner arch on the prefabricated Kloehn bow. Thinner wires on laboratory made Kloehn bows eg 1.0mm will distort and prevent the linking system described in Design Card 12B from functioning.

- The mesial of the tube is placed 3-4mm distal to the anterior open bite. **Thus the further distally the AOB extends, then the further distally will the headgear tube be placed.** This concentrates the intruding force on the maxillary buccal teeth that need to be intruded. If in doubt on this point, consult the clinician.

- Headgear tubes bought from suppliers come attached to plates intended for inserting into the acrylic. These tend to balance on the tips of the cusps, and require more bite opening and thicker buccal overlays which in turn reduces patient tolerance. It is better to make the flying headgear tube assembly in the laboratory with wire.

- The flying headgear tube is waxed in place. For patient tolerance it wants to be minimally protruding from the side of the buccal overlay. The adequacy of the path of insertion of the headgear inner bow should be tested with a piece of straight wire.

- The midline screw should be placed and the appliance should be waxed up to the previously set degree of buccal opening. A short, angled wire should be placed in the headgear tube to help the otherwise floating headgear assembly stay in the correct place in the plaster during flasking and packing.

- The appliance should be heatcured for maximum strength of reasonable thickness buccal overlays.

- In addition to a high polish on the tongue side of the appliance, the acrylic should be checked for any pimples or roughness and lightly polished on the fitting surface of the appliance.

- Very carefully check the projecting headgear tubes for any roughness mesially or distally and smooth with a hard rubber wheel.

- Fit the inner arch of the Kloehn bow to the tubes with small bayonet bends as stops at the mesial of the headgear tubes.

- The clinician will adjust the outer Kloehn bow.

Functional Component Objectives

1. Maximised intrusion of the upper buccal segment teeth that are propping the occlusion. (Intrusion and supression of growth is about 2mm).

2. Minimised retrusion and distal tipping of the upper buccal segments. (If $\underline{7|7}$ extraction is planned it is better to leave $\underline{7|7}$ in situ until the intrusive phase is completed. But if $\frac{7|7}{7|7}$ extractions are planned continue with $\overline{7|7}$ extractions from the start of treatment).

3. Minimised eruption of the lower buccal segments. (Rebuild the upper buccal overlays 3-4 months into treatment).

4. Total freedom for spontaneous vertical development of the upper and lower labial segments.

5. Reduction in the anterior open bite by differential vertical development, or suppression, of the labial and buccal segments respectively.

6. Reduction of the anterior open bite by forward mandibular hinging giving spontaneous overjet reduction of 4-6mm. This consequence is only of value in the Class II case.

7. Reduction of the lower anterior face height as a percentage of total face height by 1-2%.

   NOTE To conform with standard user convention (UK & USA) **the tubing sizes only** are shown in thousandths of an inch.

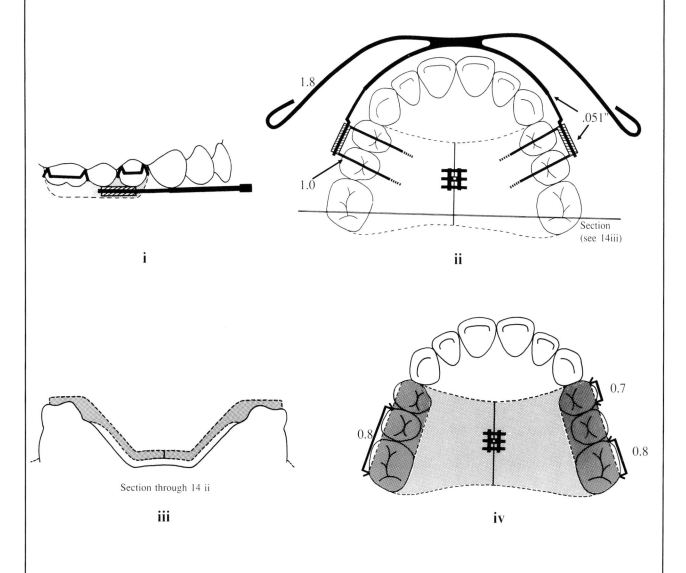

i

ii

Section through 14 ii

iii

iv

Wire size conversion mm to American Gauge) : 0.7 = 21, 0.8 = 20, 1.0 = 18, 1.5 = 15, 1.8 = 13

Clinical guidance on prescription

- **Prescribe for gummy Class II Division 1 occlusions with visible and vulnerable upper incisors and with starting overjets of less than 8-9mm.**

- Where the starting overjet is greater than 8-9mm use the systems shown in Design Cards 16 or 17.

- Look at the starting study models and bring the incisors into a position of reduced overjet. Invariably expansion of the upper buccal segments and frequently some alignment of the upper labial segment is needed with the initial use of an ELSAA appliance.

- The ELSAA appliances shown in Design Cards 4 i & ii, 5 iii & iv and 6 i & ii will most commonly be required.

- Avoid the use of anterior brackets (Design Card 4 iii & iv) **wherever possible,** since anterior brackets during the MIS phase of treatment limit the depth of the incisal capping and this predisposes towards over-uprighting of _III_.

- If anterior brackets are needed during the ELSAA phase for labial segment alignment (Design Card 4 iii & iv), then it is better to gain alignment, remove the brackets, and place a Hawley retainer prior to taking working impressions for the MIS. The Hawley retainer must, however, be worn all the time that the MIS is out of the mouth. This approach minimises the risk of decalcification on the labial surface of the incisors due to protracted wear of anterior brackets.

- More rarely **GUMMY Class II Division 2 malocclusions** may present.

- These **should be converted into Class II Division 1 malocclusions** by the use of ELSAA designs 5 i & ii. Less commonly designs 6 iii & iv may be employed.

- To compensate for secondary uprighting of _III_ during the MIS, or during the activator phase of treatment Class II Division 2 upper central incisors should be overproclined to 125°.

- It is very easy to open upper labial segment spacing in Class II Division 2 cases (ie **never extract** _4I4_ **in Class II Division 2 cases,** however crowded the case may seem), and be prepared to use anterior brackets to gather _4+4_ together. Again it is better to remove the brackets immediately prior to the MIS phase of treatment.

- **Whilst most MIS cases are preferably treated, non-extraction or with loss of** _7I7_, **upper mid-arch spacing which may be present for a variety of reasons does not contraindicate the use of the MIS.**

- The general principle is to gather any anterior spaced teeth into an upper labial segment block with an appropriate variant of ELSAA Design Card 7.

- The technician then undertakes a 'tunnel' plastering within and posterior to the localised mid-arch space. This 'tunnel' plastering blocks out the mid-arch space, and on the posterior molars fills the occlusal fissures up to the level of the tips of the cusps, as well as filling interdentally on the palatal out to the level of the maximum palatal curvature (see also page 68).

- It goes without saying that any clasping must be anterior to the gathered mid-arch space. The posterior segment is thus **controlled vertically,** but is **free to move mesially** as the anterior, tightly gripped, and acrylic enclosed labial segment is moved distally. This need for satisfactory clasping is the reason that anterior spacing is best gathered at least from _4+4_.

- In the clinical prescription of a MIS, a lateral skull film is needed to confirm the initial clinical diagnosis. A careful detailed design taking account of the factors listed above should then be undertaken.

- Upper and lower impressions and a maximum intercuspation bite are needed. It has been found quite satisfactory for the technician to open the hinge of a plane line articulator to give an adequate thickness of buccal overlay.

- The headgear (see Design Card 12A) should always be fabricated IN ADVANCE of the fit visit of the MIS, so that the clinician can concentrate on the details of finding the centre of balance of the linking system (see Design Card 12B), fitting the appliance well and instructing the child and parent. Headgear routine and pressures are described in Design Card 12A. 12-14 hours per day of headgear appliance wear is asked for. The previous ELSAA, with the screw sealed with acrylic, is worn when the MIS is out of the mouth.

- The buccal overlays usually need light equilibration.

- At subsequent visits check the cribbing and tap lightly on the incisal wire to ensure that is firmly in contact with _III_. **Marginally activate as necessary.**

See overleaf for technical guidance on construction

Functional Component Objectives

1. Intrusion of ⊥⊥⊥ relative to the resting upper lip length (gains of 2mm can be routinely expected. It is important to monitor this intrusion during treatment since overtreatment may occur relatively easily with the over-enthusiastic patient).

2. Vertical restraint of the upper buccal segments (1.8mm on 6|6 in 1 year).

3. Sagittal restraint of the maxilla. (Superimposed tracings have in some cases shown a distal movement of 1-2mm of the posterior nasal spine where the headgear hook is too close to the ear).

4. 'En masse' distal movement of the upper buccal segments (maximised by extraction of 7|7 , minimised by the presence of 7|7 . Either situation may be clinically appropriate).

5. Some uprighting of the very proclined ⊥⊥⊥ (ie where ⊥⊥⊥ are greater than 115° at the start of the MIS phase of treatment).

6. Minimised uprighting of ⊥⊥⊥ where the starting inclination is less than 115° (This is **the most common case,** which will therefore require **the deepest feasible incisal capping and a curved goalpost wire on ⊥⊥⊥).**

7. Spontaneous overjet reduction (7-8mm) partially due to uprighting of ⊥⊥⊥ (10°) and partially due to forward mandibular hinging (worth 3-4mm at ⊤⊤⊤ tips). The degree of favourable forward mandibular hinging is however quite variable from patient to patient.

8. Finally and most importantly, a maximised improvement in the position of visible and vulnerable upper incisors, by their intrusion, in Class II Division 1 patients having a gummy smile.

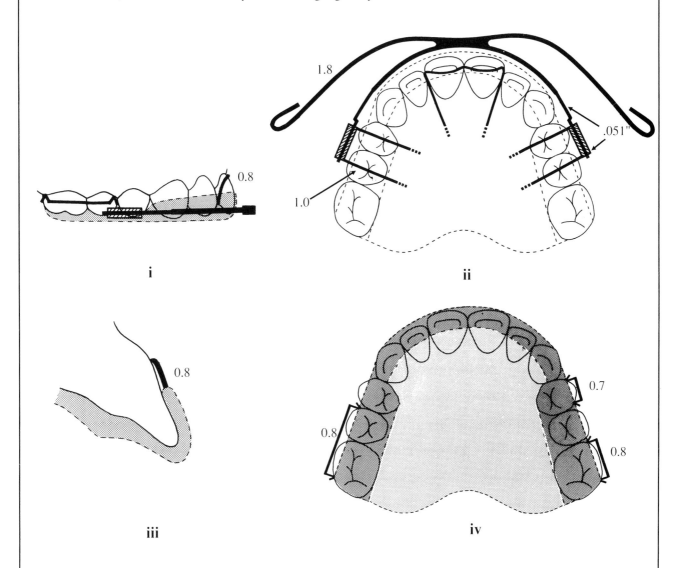

i

ii

iii

iv

Wire size conversion (mm to American Gauge) : 0.7 = 21, 0.8 = 20, 1.0 = 18, 1.8 = 13

Technical guidance on construction

- Unlike the Buccal Intrusion Splint there is NO wax relief of the palate.

- The upper and lower working models are articulated on a hinged articulator in the maximum intercuspation bite obtained by the clinician.

- The upper working model is first examined from the point of view of any plastering relief of the teeth (the majority of cases do not require this)
  Any interdental spaces between the incisors are plastered out.
  If there is significant buccal segment spacing to close, then 'tunnel' plastering will be needed posteriorly, to allow the teeth distal to the gap to move mesially.
  The object of 'tunnel' plastering is to control the posterior teeth VERTICALLY but to allow the teeth **distal to the mid-arch space** to move mesially within the splint.
  The fissures of the molars, and occasionally a premolar, are plastered leaving the tips of the cusp just clear of the plaster.
  The palatal interdental embrasures are filled out to the line of the palatal surfaces of the molars.

- The bite should be opened just enough (1.5-2.0mm) for adequate strength of acrylic heat-cured buccal overlays. The buccal overlays MUST NOT BREAK UP, **but the patient must be able to tolerate the degree of bite opening.**

- Cribbing choice is optional dependent on the needs of the case. Most MIS appliances are for non-extraction or 7|7 extraction cases. Double cribs (0.8mm wire) on 65|56 or 6E|E6 are usually most appropriate. If tunnel plastering has been undertaken, 4|4 cribs may be needed. **Transdental crib embrasure plastering is obligatory.**

- A curved goalpost-shaped piece of wire is placed on 1|1, to minimise palatal tipping of 1|1. The transverse part of the wire wants to be as close to the gingival margins of 1|1 as the interdental papilla will permit. A V-shaped compensation is usually made to allow for the interdental papilla.

- The flying headgear tube component is as described in the BIS technical guidance. The mesial of the tube is lined up with the tip of the cusp of 4|4. The inner bow of the Kloehn bow is very short, stiff and inevitably has some divergence. If however the headgear tubes are placed too parallel, the mesial of the tube will aggravate the corner of the patient's mouth. A compromise is sought using 2 straight pieces of thick wire, one in each tube to line up the headgear tubing. The tubing should be set as far **into the acrylic overlay as possible,** consistent with the ability to insert the Kloehn whisker.

- The appliance is then waxed up to the clinician's outline. The buccal overlays **should not extend buccally past the tips of the buccal cusps.** The incisal capping must be **as deep as possible** consistent with a path of entry that will give full seating of the appliance. The bite opening should be checked.

- **The appliance should be invested and heat cured.** It is not feasible to make adequately strong, thin, non-bulky incisal capping with an autopolymerised acrylic. A short angled wire should be placed in the headgear tube to help the otherwise floating headgear assembly stay in the correct place in the plaster during flaskig and packing.

- The appliance should be highly polished on the tongue side, and checked for pimples and roughness on the fit surface, before lightly polishing the fitting surface. Check the incisal capping for interdental spicules of acrylic and excessive undercuts.

- **In particular the ends of the headgear tubing must be as smoothed as possible.**

- Fit the Kloehn bow using a **small** incisally directed bayonet bend, to bring the inner arch of the bow level with the tips of the cusps. It may be necessary to remove a small portion of the inner bow stiffening tubing due to the short inter-tube distance. At the appropriate mark the tubing is scored around its diameter with a small sharp edged disc and it can then be rotated off. The Kloehn inner bow stiffening tubing can then act as a stop.

- The clinician will adjust the Kloehn outer bow.

Functional Component Objectives

1. Intrusion of 1|1 relative to the resting upper lip length (gains of 2mm can be routinely expected. It is important to monitor this intrusion during treatment since overtreatment may occur relatively easily with the over-enthusiastic patient).

2. Vertical restraint of the upper buccal segments (1.8mm on 6|6 in 1 year).

3. Sagittal restraint of the maxilla. (Superimposed tracings have in some cases shown a distal movement of 1-2mm of the posterior nasal spine where the headgear hook is too close to the ear).

4. 'En masse' distal movement of the upper buccal segments (maximised by extraction of 7|7 , minimised by the presence of 7|7 . Either situation may be clinically appropriate).

5. Some uprighting of the very proclined 1|1 (ie where 1|1 are greater than 115° at the start of the MIS phase of treatment).

6. Minimised uprighting of 1|1 where the starting inclination is less than 115° (This is **the most common case,** which will therefore require **the deepest feasible incisal capping and a curved goalpost wire on 1|1).**

7. Spontaneous overjet reduction (7-8mm) partially due to uprighting of 1|1 (10°) and partially due to forward mandibular hinging (worth 3-4mm at 1|1 tips). The degree of favourable forward mandibular hinging is however quite variable from patient to patient.

8. Finally and most importantly, a maximised improvement in the position of visible and vulnerable upper incisors, by their intrusion, in Class II Division 1 patients having a gummy smile.

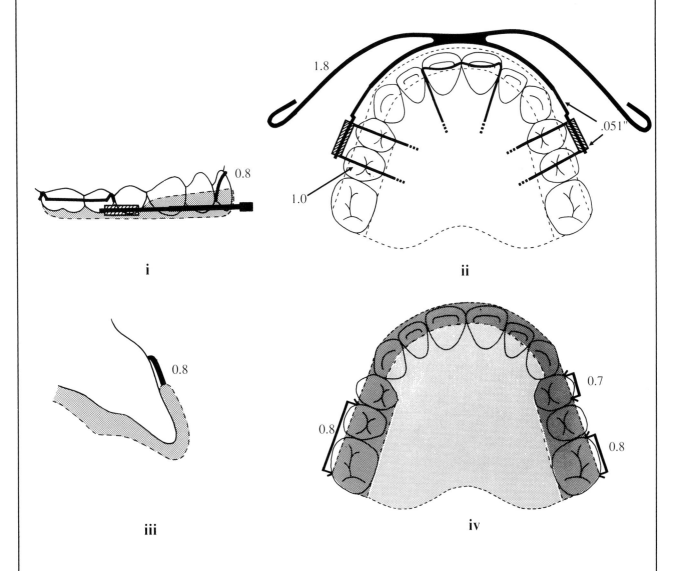

i

ii

iii

iv

Wire size conversion (mm to American Gauge) : 0.7 = 21, 0.8 = 20, 1.0 = 18, 1.8 = 13

Clinical guidance on prescription

- **Prescribe for severe, gummy Class II Division 1 occlusions with visible and vulnerable upper incisors, starting overjets of 8-18mm and AVERAGE FRANKFURT MANDIBULAR PLANE ANGLES.**

- This group of malocclusions can also be treated using the intrusive activator (see Design Card 17).

- The MIS plus Clark type traction plate appliance system is probably the most 'patient tolerable' of the functional appliance systems **that will cope** with severe Class II Division 1 malocclusions.

- The MIS plus Clark type lower produces enhanced increments of mandibular growth, though less predictably than those produced by the intrusive activator, particularly in the doubtful patient cooperator.

- The MIS plus Clark type lower, is however a more wearable system than the intrusive activator and does not muffle speech.

- The MIS plus Clark type lower is particularly appropriate for **the very enthusiastic, highly cooperative patient,** and in these circumstances will induce 3-4mm of pogonial advance in one year.

- In this type of case a reduced overbite and overjet can be achieved in 1 year from a starting 15-16mm overjet.

- At this point continue maximum appliance wear (eg 12-14 hours) for 3-4 months before reducing to night-time wear only. Night-time wear should be continued **until facial growth is complete.**

- If a period of fixed appliance work (6-9 months, during the 12-14 years of age period) is needed, then light Class II traction is indicated to gently stabilise the occlusal changes that have been induced. Similar mechanics can be continued into nocturnally worn upper and lower Hawley retainers.

- Whilst this retention regime may sound both complex and protracted, the reasons for it are readily appreciated by previously facially handicapped patients who have become facially handsome, and will have avoided the trauma, possible morbidity and occasional uncertainty of an orthognathic surgical treatment.

- It also gives an early (9-12 years) adjustment of facial handicap and the possibility of a balanced social development during the important teenage years.

- The upper appliance design is identical to the MIS on Design Card 15, but with the addition of a 'concorde' hook to the Kloehn bow.

- Contrary to popular belief **it is possible to make stable retentive lower appliances for most cases.** This does however require clinical and laboratory attention to detail.

- In the design of the lower appliance **use every undercut that is available both anteriorly and posteriorly.** Much will depend on whether there is a mixed or full permanent dentiton. $\overline{DC|CD}$ have little vertical anchorage value; $\overline{E|E}$ can be excellent; $\overline{54|45}$ are good if well erupted; $\overline{3|3}$ if fully erupted can be very valuable and $\overline{6|6}$ are usually satisfactory from the age of 9 years. With two appliances in the mouth, tolerance is improved if, consistent with anchorage and retention, the lower appliance can be kept as small as feasible. Lower cribs can be made in 0.7mm wire to improve the flexible engagement of undercuts.

- The semi-fitted lower labial bow (which does not enter the interdental embrasures) combines with the posterior undercuts to give added vertical retention.

- The lingual hook for the anterior elastic is made in soft stainless steel wire and wants to be as small as possible, consistent with function.

- Good quality impressions should be obtained and cast quickly. A maximum intercuspation bite is required since the forward mandibular displacement is elastic induced. The appliance fit visit should be arranged within 2 weeks of the impressions being taken.

- The headgear should be fabricated at the impression visit (Design Card 12A) so that the clinician can then concentrate on the appliance fit, patient instructions and motivation of the patient at the appliance fit visit.

- A graded series of 2-3 packets of elastics should be given to induce up to 200 grams of forward mandibular displacement. The 5/16" medium wall extra-oral elastics can eventually be accomodated and have been found to be clinically successful. Headgear elastics should be graded from 75 to 400+ grams as was previously described for Design Card 12A.

See overleaf for technical guidance on construction

THE MIS with 'concorde' whisker & Clark type lower traction plate.

FUNCTIONAL
APPLIANCE
DESIGN CARD

16

Functional Component Objectives

1. See Design Card 15, for objectives 1-6 & 8 which apply similarly to this appliance.

2. Use of the headgear stabilised maxillary dentition as an anchorage base for an elastic propelled, forward displacement of the mandible and mandibular dentition (via the 'concorde' whisker).

3. Maximised increments of the condylar growth mechanism.

4. Minimised proclination of the lower incisors.

5. Reduction of large overjets (9-18mm) and the achievement of a Class I incisor relationship with minimised uprighting of the upper incisors.

6. Maximised improvement in facial retrognathia.

7. A relaxed lips together seal without conscious effort and with reduced visibility of the upper incisors.

8. In summary **treatment of severe gummy Class II Division 1 occlusions with average face heights.**

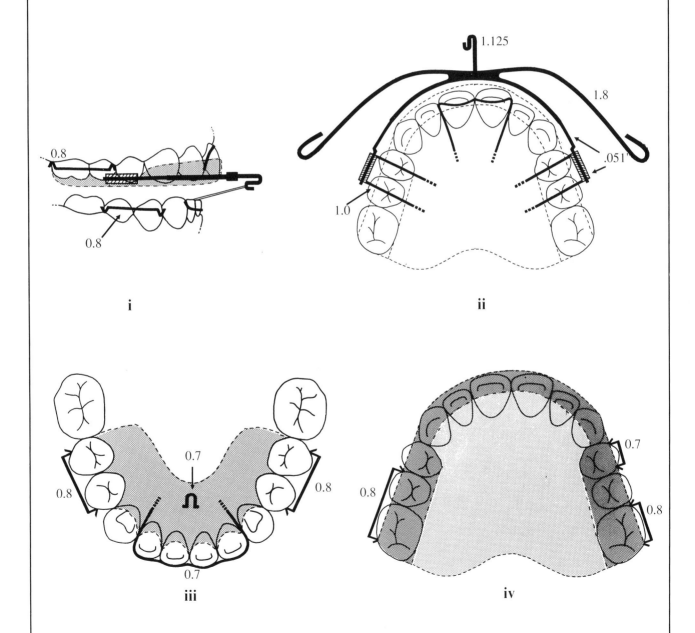

i

ii

iii

iv

Wire size conversion (mm to American Gauge) : 0.7 = 21, 0.8 = 20, 1.0 = 18, 1.125 = 17, 1.8 = 13

THE MIS with 'concorde' whisker &
Clark type lower traction plate
(continued)

16

Technical guidance on construction

- The upper appliance construction details are identical to those on Design Card 15 with the addition of the 'concorde' hook to a factory manufactured Kloehn headgear bow.

  NOTE : The term 'EOT (extra oral traction) whisker' is used in the United Kingdom instead of 'Kloehn bow'. At an earlier stage of development in the United Kingdom these bows were fabricated in the laboratory, but this produced a bow or whisker which was not rigid enough for this type of mechanics. The name for this modified whisker originally derived from the downward droop of the thinner diameter anterior hook which in profile, was compared to the drooping nose-cone of the Concorde aeroplane. The use of factory manufactured Kloehn bows and thicker section wires have remedied this problem but the 'concorde' name remains.

- An anterior 1.125mm wire is soldered to the Kloehn bow. By arrangement with the clinician this is either left straight for the clinician to adapt or bent up to a previously agreed shape in the laboratory.

- On the **lower working model** any soft tissue lingual undercuts should be plastered out.

- For the lower appliance study the tooth undercut availability and decide whether a retentive appliance is feasible. If there is doubt, telephone the clinician. In doubtful retentive situations the final selection of the pattern of cribbing is best left to an informed technician.

- 0.8mm wires should be used for cribs wherever possible, since it reduces crib breakage significantly.

- Use double cribs whenever possible. Try to avoid two wires passing through the same embrasure if possible, but this may be needed at the insertion of the labial bow.

- Fabricate the lower labial bow in 0.7mm wire. It should be placed as far gingivally as the interdental papillae permit, and should hug the labial surface of all the incisors in a series of flowing mini-curves. Do not go too far interdentally since the inevitable high spots will prevent the wire from being snugged down on the labial with a maximum engagement of undercut. Also interdental undercut engagement can harm the interdental papillae and makes the appliance less tolerable to the child.

- The lower lingual hook for elastic traction to the 'concorde' bow is fabricated in soft 0.7mm stainless steel wire and is left projecting vertically so that it will stabilise the wire during flasking and packing the appliance. The hook is flattened into its final position after finishing.

- Since the upper appliance can only be satisfactorily constructed in heat cured acrylic, it is advantageous to heat cure the lower also.

Functional Component Objectives

1. See Design Card 15, for objectives 1-6 & 8 which apply similarly to this appliance.

2. Use of the headgear stabilised maxillary dentition as an anchorage base for an elastic propelled, forward displacement of the mandible and mandibular dentition (via the 'concorde' whisker).

3. Maximised increments of the condylar growth mechanism.

4. Minimised proclination of the lower incisors.

5. Reduction of large overjets (9-18mm) and the achievement of a Class I incisor relationship with minimised uprighting of the upper incisors.

6. Maximised improvement in facial retrognathia.

7. A relaxed lips together seal without conscious effort and with reduced visibility of the upper incisors.

8. In summary **treatment of severe gummy Class II Division 1 occlusions with average face heights.**

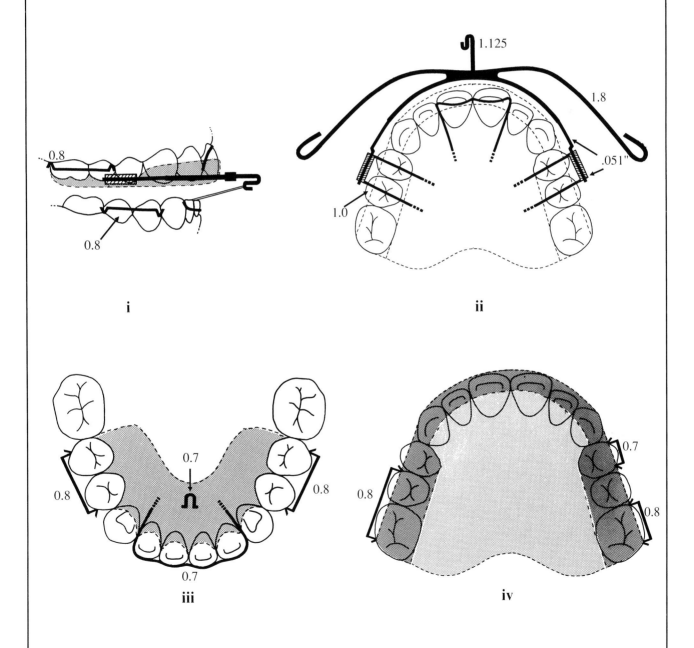

i

ii

iii

iv

Wire size conversion (mm to American Gauge) : 0.7 = 21, 0.8 = 20, 1.0 = 18, 1.125 = 17, 1.8 = 13

Clinical guidance on prescription

- **Prescribe for LONG-FACED (ie high FMPA), severe, gummy, Class II Division 1 occlusions, where ⊥⊥⊥ are overvisible during resting and expressive lip behaviour.**

- The intrusive activator is **also valuable** in the treatment of **averageFMPA,** severe, gummy, Class II Division 1 occlusions (see also Design Card 16).

- The comments on Design Card 15 concerning any preliminary maxillary arch expansion with ELSAA appliances and the management of any upper arch interdental spacing are all appropriate to the design and use of the intrusive activator.

- A reasonably aligned lower arch and lower labial segment is also needed for the satisfactory prescription of the intrusive activator. The approach to this has already been outlined in the clinical guidance notes for Design Cards 8 and 9. If alignment of the lower labial segment was indicated, then this would be initiated at the beginning of the ELSAA phase of treatment.

- The intrusive activator muffles speech and is less tolerable for protracted wear than medium opening activators. **It is, to date, the only satisfactory, predictable and relatively rapid, orthodontic treatment modality for the management of severe (up to 18mm of overjet), gummy (5-6mm of gum visible during expressive behaviour), long-faced Class II Division 1 malocclusons.**

- Since these malocclusions have substantial treatment need and the only satisfactory appliance system 'to date' is difficult to tolerate, **it is most important that the appliance is made as acceptable as possible to the patient.**

- The bite for the first appliance should be 4-5mm forward only and quite close; ie not more than 2-3mm open.

- It is critical that the lingual and palatal acrylic is **as thin as possible** to obtain maximum space for the tongue.

- To aid the introduction to the whole appliance system, the headgear is fitted (Design Card 12A & B), but the intra-oral appliance only, is worn for the first week, before starting the headgear in the second week.

- The fused ELSAA appliance is, of course, worn during all meals and when the intrusive activator is out of the mouth.

- This appliance should be relatively passive by 4 months when a more active (6mm advance and 4mm open) bite should be obtained for the second appliance.

- It may be possible to cut a small anterior breathing slit in this second appliance which will have more vertical space above the lower incisal capping.

- The second appliance will become passive at 9-10 months when a third appliance should be made. This third appliance should overcorrect the slight Class II into a Class III incisal relationship with an active bite of 1-2mm of reverse overjet.

- If the bite on the second appliance has been sufficiently open vertically, there may be adequate acrylic for the technician to use a fret saw to seperate the upper from the lower. The irregular joins are smoothed, and the patient postures forward for the desired mild Class III incisor bite. The two halves are sealed with wax prior to fusing with auto-polymerising acrylic in the laboratory. This may be an alternative to making a third appliance.

- Whilst three intrusive activators may seem an expensive way of treating a case, these malocclusions are so challenging, and so unsatisfactorily handled with other techniques, that the cost is justified.

- Treatment times are frequently as little as a year for 15-16mm overjets.

- The retention approach is similar to that outlined in the clinical guidance for Design Card 16.

- Particularly for the very long-faced dolichocephalic patient, an intrusive headgear component should be kept going on a night-time only basis for a few years.

- If the intrusive activator is used for average FMPA cases, then the treatment **must** be reviewed cephalometrically to ensure that neither excessive intrusion of upper incisors nor excessive sagittal arrest of the maxillary dentition is occurring.

- If enough forward checking of the maxilla has occurred **then stopping the headgear,** but **continuing with the activator may be indicated.**

See overleaf for technical guidance on construction

Functional Component Objectives

1. See Design Card 15, for objectives 1-6 & 8 which apply similarly to this appliance.

2. See Design Card 16, for objectives 3-7 which apply similarly to this appliance.

3. Suppression of the vertical development of $\overline{7654|4567}$ **as well as** suppression of the vertical development of $\underline{7654|4567}$. In most cases $\frac{7|7}{7|7}$ are still unerupted during the period of treatment.

4. A more sure induction of forward mandibular hinging than using Design Card 16.

5. The reduction of excess lower anterior face height as a percentage of total face height.

6. Reduction of the inadequacy of soft tissue cover of the lower anterior face.

7. The satisfactory treatment of severe long faced gummy Class II Division 1 malocclusion.

   NOTE : Progressive cephalometric assessment should be undertaken 6-9 months into treatment **to confirm whether the headgear should be continued, or stopped** to avoid overtreating the sagittal, OR the vertical, restraint of the maxillary dentition.

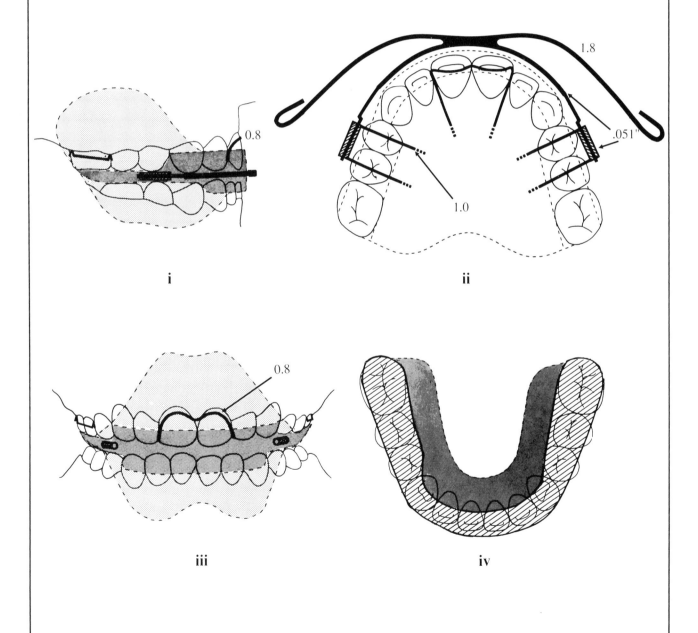

i

ii

iii

iv

Wire size conversion (mm to American Gauge) : 0.8 = 20, 1.0 = 18, 1.8 = 13

Technical guidance on construction

- The upper and lower working models are articulated on a plane line or plasterless articulator from the front, **with the anterior teeth facing towards the pillar of the articulator.** Set and RECORD the vertical dimension.

- The working models should then be removed from the articulator for occlusal plastering.

- The intention of the initial plastering of the working models is to allow slight bucco-lingual, and mesio-distal, minor adjustment of premolars and lower molars, whilst **preventing any eruption** of buccal segment teeth.

- The occlusal fissures of the upper molars and premolars are plastered just up to the level of the tips of the cusps. The tips of the cusps must be just visible. Plaster interdentally on the palatal but NOT covering the greatest palatal curvature of each buccal segment tooth.

- On the lower working model the occlusal surfaces of the premolars and molars are plastered similarly, but additionally the interdental lingual embrasures are plastered out. The lower cheek teeth will thus be enclosed in an 'L' of acrylic which is in contact with the tips of the cusps and the lingual surfaces.

- Minimal plastering of irregular lower incisors may be required, similar to that given in the technical guidance for the MOA-Palatal, Design Card 8.

- The wirework is identical to that described for the MIS, Design Card 15, with appropriate embrasure plastering of the cribs.

- The upper wax work is completed and the articulator closed to ensure that the bite has not been propped open.

- Adapt one sheet of wax to the lower outline required and thicken in the lingual area by a further 1mm.

- A second trial closure is needed to see that there is no gagging of the bite. After this has been adjusted, the upper and lower waxes are sealed together with an interstitial roll of warmed wax.

- It is most important to carefully smooth, fill, thin and polish the wax-work to minimise acrylic finishing, and to ensure later minimal thickness of acrylic.

- The appliance is cured on both working models which need to be **invested in a deep activator flask.**

- Grind away excess plaster from the upper and lower models before investing.

- The upper and lower working models are settled, upper incisors down, into a bed of plaster in the deep half of the flask.

- Flasking is then completed and the appliance packed with **clear heat cured acrylic.**

- The appliance must be well finished and highly polished, particularly on the lingual. The objective is to have the lingual acrylic as thin as is feasible, from the point of view of strength and finishing. The lingual flanges must have rounded, not sharp margins.

- The headgear tubes should be smoothed, and the inner arch of a Kloehn bow should be fitted to the intrusive activator.

- The outer bow is left for the clinician to adjust as in Design Card 12B.

Functional Component Objectives

1. See Design Card 15, for objectives 1-6 & 8 which apply similarly to this appliance.

2. See Design Card 16, for objectives 3-7 which apply similarly to this appliance.

3. Suppression of the vertical development of $\overline{7654|4567}$ **as well as** suppression of the vertical development of $\underline{7654|4567}$. In most cases $\frac{7|7}{7|7}$ are still unerupted during the period of treatment.

4. A more sure induction of forward mandibular hinging than using Design Card 16.

5. The reduction of excess lower anterior face height as a percentage of total face height.

6. Reduction of the inadequacy of soft tissue cover of the lower anterior face.

7. The satisfactory treatment of severe long faced gummy Class II Division 1 malocclusion.

   NOTE : Progressive cephalometric assessment should be undertaken 6-9 months into treatment **to confirm whether the headgear should be continued, or stopped** to avoid overtreating the sagittal, OR the vertical, restraint of the maxillary dentition.

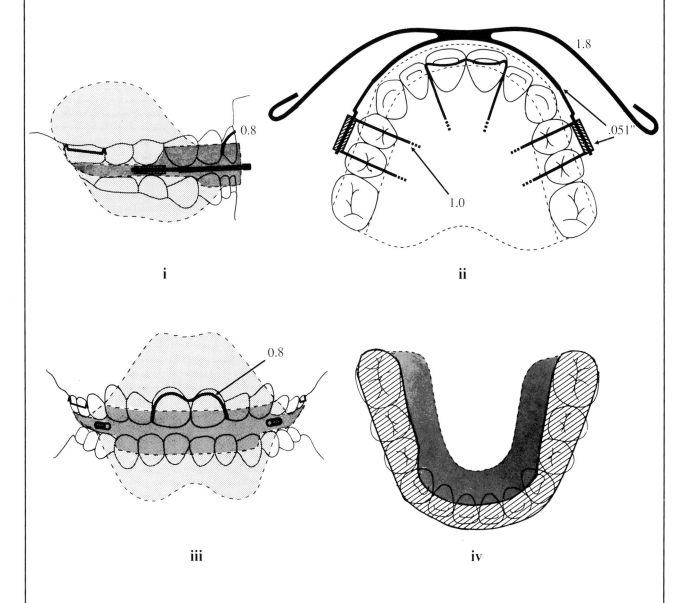

i

ii

iii

iv

Wire size conversion (mm to American Gauge) : 0.8 = 20, 1.0 = 18, 1.8 = 13

CHAPTER FIVE

THE HERBST ACRYLIC SPLINT
DESIGN CARD 18

There are a small percentage of patients with severe, facially handicapping Class II malocclusions who are unable for a variety of psycho-social reasons to cooperate with a functional appliance. The size of this small group declines with increasing clinical functional appliance experience and skill. Finding the right appliance for the reluctant child is not dissimilar to presenting just the right fly to a reluctant trout. There are, however, days when even the most skilled fishermen return empty handed. When a child is in the mixed dentition, and is unable, despite every effort, to cooperate; then the treatment should be abandoned and the child issued with a sports guard. A fresh functional appliance approach, bearing in mind the previous lessons, may well be successful eighteen months later. However for the early maturing 12-14 year old, 18 months later may be too late for a Class II functional appliance to work. Frequently the situation is a cause of great worry within the family and has substantial consequences for the longterm emotional, social and educational well-being of the patient.

At this point procedures which carry more risk need to be considered. For this group of patients with substantial skeletal II malocclusions there are two alternatives; the Herbst acrylic splint or orthognathic surgery.

ORTHOGNATHIC   SURGERY

Over a period of years, many orthognathic patients have been seen who have been treated by various oral and maxillo-facial surgeons. There are a number of facial dysplasias which unlike severe facial retrognathias, are beyond the scope of orthodontic treatment. **Many orthognathic surgical results have been seen which are a delight to the clinical observer and the patient,** and which give a comprehensive and full treatment of the underlying facial dysplasia and occlusal problem. For these cases a harmonious integration of pre-surgical occlusal orthodontic treatment and orthognathic surgery is generally required. There are however many patients and parents who are quite unwilling to entertain orthognathic surgery as a solution for their very retrognathic children. Also it has to be recognised **that the morbidity associated with orthognathic surgery is substantial, frequently unacknowledged, and that a small, but significant percentage of cases go seriously wrong.** It is within this context that the problems associated with the Herbst acrylic splint have to be set.

THE   HERBST   APPLIANCE

The Herbst 'bite jumping' appliance was first reported by Emil Herbst in the early 1900's. The appliance caused the mandible to be held in a forward position by a hinged piston which entered a hinged tube fixed to the maxillary dentition. After some initial popularity the appliance fell into decline until rescued by W. Pancherz in the 1970's. Much of Pancherz's early work revolved around an appliance which had very stiff bands on $\overline{4|4}$, which were connected by a lingual bar. Onto the buccal of these $\overline{4|4}$ bands, were soldered the mandibular pistons. This appliance system demonstrated a valuable correction of Class II buccal occlusions but an unwanted substantial proclination of lower incisors. This degree of proclination of the lower incisors would have been theoretically predictable to a conventionally trained orthodontist. Additionally it was very difficult to fabricate the very thick tape (0.175") that was required to prevent the lower first premolar bands from shearing under the thrust of the pistons. Further development of the appliance by R.P. Howe and later J.A. McNamara resulted in the initially fully bonded, but later removable **Herbst acrylic splint appliance.** This bonded appliance should now be included in the armamentarium of all clinicians interested in the treatment of serious Class II malocclusion, in the permanent   dentition.

MAXILLARY SPLINT DESIGN & ACRYLIC COVERAGE

The upper splint carries the hinged tube that receives the hinged piston which displaces the mandible forward. When the mouth is opened the piston extends from the tube and re-enters the tube on mouth closure. If the piston/tube combination is too short, the piston falls out as the patient opens his mouth. If the piston is long with a shortish tube, then on closure the end of the piston emerges from the back of the tube and can produce quite severe cheek ulceration. One therefore seeks **as long a piston/tube combination as is possible with the mouth closed.** The upper and lower hinges are placed respectively as far distally and mesially as feasible. There are, however, natural limits to this. In the upper (for the lower see the next section) the hinge of the tube is placed on the disto-buccal of the upper first molar. If the hinge is placed on the upper second molar it will give serious ulceration problems over the coronoid process.

The upper buccal segments need to expand as the Class II correction is completed. This can be achieved by having a 'U' loop in the transpalatal wire. This heavy transpalatal wire is relieved from the palate by 5.0mm. A **gentle** squeeze of the 'U' loop, with a degree of activation that is felt rather than seen, ensures the maintenance of a normal bucco-lingual relationship as the Class II sagittal correction takes place. If a rapid maxillary expansion screw is soldered into position it gives a bulky and unhygienic appliance.

A variety of designs have been tried. A full arch (with 654|456 palatal, occlusal and buccal coverage and 321|123 palatal and incisal tip coverage) does give bodily control of 1|1 and no induction of upper arch spacing. Upper arch expansion is NOT possible and IF $3+3$ CAPPING SHOULD LEAK the decalcification of the incisors **is visible and unpleasant.**

The buccal segment capping has also been extended forward to include the maxillary canines (either fully or just on the palatal). If this coverage is on the palatal only, the bonding may fail on one of the canine teeth and caries may penetrate to dentine if this is not spotted. Frequently, 3|3 are buccally or mesially placed with a small span of gum between the mesial of 4|4 and the distal of 3|3. Inevitably, if this span of gum is bridged by acrylic and is compressed by composite as it sets, it will result in a severe desquamative gingivitis under this small saddle of composite. Wherever there is a break in the dental continuity of the arch with acrylic capping mesial and distal to the space, then the break or saddle **must be linked by the bar of wire only** and not bridged by acrylic to avoid compression of the gum by composite and induction of a severe gingivitis in this region. Inclusion of 3|3 in the acrylic coverage of the buccal segment is generally not advised UNLESS 3|3 are perfectly lined up with 654|456 .

The most satisfactory general maxillary acrylic outline is coverage of 654|456, with a wire spur to control 7|7 vertically if needed. The forward mandibular displacement is thus **only resisted by the upper buccal segments.** Space opens distal to 3|3 as 654|456 are moved distally. For this reason 0.9mm tubes on a supporting squared off 'U' of 0.8mm wire are placed in the buccal overlay in the first premolar region. This is the guiding buccal tube for a free sliding anterior wire that is used to gather up any spacing in the labial segments. The labial wire can be either a stiff round 0.8mm wire with a forward hook activated by elastics that are changed by the patient; or a thick section rectangular nickel-titanium wire inserted into a few anterior brackets and activated by linked chain. **Since the maximum overjet is required for maximum mandibular advance** via the re-activated pistons, the operator should **be cautious about an over-enthusiastic early closure of anterior spacing.** Generally, anterior space closure is undertaken during the settling period when the pistons and lower splint have just been discarded. The timing of management is discussed below.

MANDIBULAR SPLINT DESIGN & ACRYLIC COVERAGE

A major concern in the lower arch is the probability of excessive protrusion of the lower incisors. This tendency is minimised by the lower incisor capping (3-4 mm deep), which when the composite has set, has a very substantial degree of bodily control of 321|123. The buccal overlay extends to the distal of the first molar. Do not attempt to cover 7|7 if present, either partially or fully, **but rely on a distal wire prong set into the acrylic to control 7|7 vertically.** The mandibular piston swivel wants to be soldered as far forwards as possible. Effectively this is on the mesio-buccal of 4|4.

VERTICAL SPLINT DESIGN (Depth of the capping)

The vertical extention of the capping of the upper and lower splint is a matter of substantial clinical importance. All acrylic gingival margins have a fine champhered edge that is placed 0.5-1mm from the patient's gingival margins on the working model. Historically the clinician was most concerned with the splint staying in place. To this end the first splints were made as deep as was gingivally feasible. The gingival margins of the casts were lightly scolloped to facilitate this. There was almost an element of snap fit as the splints were tried on. It is not possible **to fully clear** the gingival margins of the composite **as the splint is bonded.** Removal of the early splints after 6-8 months of often very successful occlusal therapy, revealed the worst extensive desquamative spontaneous haemorrhaging gingivitis the author had seen. Whilst this superficially healed very quickly (2-3 weeks) with the most florid features disappearing in 2-3 days, these early experiences resulted in significant acrylic heat-cured splint modification.

The opposite problem was then encountered with there being an inadequate surface area of acrylic to stop the splint lifting at the composite/acrylic interface. This has been overcome by using a small inverted cone bur on the inner surface of the finished splint to cut a line of opposing undercuts on the buccal and lingual. The inner surface of the splint is also 'conditioned' after it has been tried in the mouth by wiping it out after cleaning, using an acrylic monomer.

CLINICAL WORKING RECORDS

Quality upper and lower working impressions should be obtained and cast without delay to obtain maximum accuracy of the working models. A bite should be obtained which is 3-4mm forward and open by 4 mm buccally. The opening is most important to gain enough (but not excessive) space for the buccal overlay acrylic. The technician should not need to alter the vertical dimension screw on the plane line articulator. The wax bite should have a 'buccal window' so that the precise degree of opening can be visualised.

The amount that the bite is taken forward is less critical since if the bite is under-activated, then the pistons can be easily advanced (see Clinical Management). The most important point to ALWAYS REMEMBER is that this patient is by definition a previously recalcitrant patient who has been persuaded into wearing a complex, sometimes difficult appliance and who should be coaxed gently into the initial, potentially awkward stages of this very effective appliance system.

BONDING THE SPLINT

The appeal of the Herbst appliance to many patients is that it takes away the need for patient cooperation. A number of previously failed functional appliance cooperators have said what a relief this is to them not to be able to remove the appliance. Therefore, with all its problems of caries through leakage and the possible induction of a significant gingivitis, the appliance system should initially be considered as a bonded rather than a removable system. **The management of the bonded appliance system should be subject to the protocol outlined below.**

A LIGHT ACTIVATED NON-VISCOUS BONDING AGENT (eg Heliosit orthodontic) should be used rather than a chemically activated composite. Chemically activated composites give inadequate working time. Since the appliance can fail at the bonding visit, **good preparation for the visit and a practice dry run with the dental surgery assistants is worthwhile.** Two assistants are needed so that one can prepare materials and pass these whilst the other dental surgery assistant concentrates single mindedly on keeping the operative field bone dry and helping with the curing light. **The need for a totally dry bonding field cannot be stressed too strongly.** Anti-sialogogues are rarely needed.

- Remove the pistons from the lower splint and place the now 'individualised pistons' in separate left and right packets in the patients model box since the piston system will not be coupled up for another week or two. It is possible for the pistons to be colour coded.

- TIGHTEN DOWN the upper screw holding the sleeve, since the rima oris of most patients is too small to allow easy access to the maxillary screw after the upper splint has been bonded.

- Try both splints in and check the occlusion. Adjust as needed.

- Pass the splints to the chairside assistant to clean, dry and 'condition' the fit surface with acrylic monomer.

- Use a tiny piece of adhesive plaster to stick the hinged tube to the occluso-buccal of the maxillary splint so that it does not flap about during bonding.

- Each arch should be prepared separately and bonded separately but at the same visit.

- Since the lower is more difficult **it is worthwhile bonding the upper splint first.**

- Speed is important as well as having everything planned and to hand since there are very large areas of teeth to be polished, etched, washed off and dried.

- Use a liquid rather than a gel etchent. Etch the buccal, palatal and cuspal tips liberally, with relatively little etch entering the occlusal fissures.

- A protracted etch time 2-2.5 minutes results from the time taken to get round all the teeth.

- It is most important that leakage does not occur from failing to etch the periphery of the whole splint.

- Isolate the arches using long curved buccal cotton wool rolls containing a plastic stiffener.

- Use long, soft, cotton wool rolls (broken at the correct length) sub-lingually, to pack the floor of the mouth. Do this for the upper arch bond-up as well, since it serves as a practice run for the lower and enables the operator to see the efficacy of the saliva ejector and the rate of flooding of the lower cotton wool rolls.

- **Do not seal any of the etched teeth** either in the upper or the lower.

- Gently overload the upper splint with unset low viscosity composite - there must be excess bonding agent but it wants to be minimised. There must not be any voids between the acrylic and the patient's enamel, since this will cause substantial enamel cavitation.

- **Make sure the cotton wool rolls are held buccally out of the way** and seat the upper splint to the position obtained when the splint was tried in the mouth.

- **With the clinician holding the splint firmly and not shifting his grip**, get the dental assistant to initiate the bonding agent set with the fibre optic light.

- It needs practice with a dry run to see how long (10, 15 or 20 seconds) is required to have the bonding material **rubbery but not set.** This is difficult to get absolutely right.

- **Still without shifting the clinician's grip** pick off the readily accessible excess composite.

- Fully set the rest of the composite making sure that each surface is approached with the fibre optic light from several directions.

- **Give the patient a good rest before restarting the whole procedure for the lower.**

- Sit the patient much MORE UPRIGHT FOR THE LOWER SPLINT BONDING since this helps to control posterior sublingual wetting.

- The bonding of the upper splint will have given the operator and assistant a preview of any dry field problems in the lower.

- The sequence for the lower is similar to that outlined above for the upper.

- Total desiccation of all etched surfaces covered by the splint is vital.

- Make especially sure, both buccally AND LINGUALLY, that the cotton wool rolls are not trapped by the edge of the splint when it is being fully seated.

- Again be very sure to hold the splint down firmly without shifting the finger grip whilst the initial set, trimming of excess bonding agent and completion of set are undertaken.

- Check the occlusion in the protrusive and retrusive bite and lightly adjust if needed.

The step by step detailed approach has been enumerated since the whole success of this valuable clinical tool can be lost by repeated loosening of either of the splints. Once the splint fails (either by loosening or by failure of the soldering of the plunger), then it must be fully removed, together with all of the interstitial and occlusal bonding agent. This is time-consuming, not easy and often promotes a brisk gingival bleed. One to two weeks of intensive oral hygiene and the stopping of appliance wear need to pass before the splint can be rebonded. It therefore pays to take detailed care in the initial bond-up. **This splint bonding visit should be arranged when the clinician is fresh, has plenty of time, has the skilled assistance of two dental surgery assistants and cannot be hassled.**

MANAGEMENT IMMEDIATELY AFTER SPLINT BONDING

Many patients find the extended splint bonding visit quite wearing. If the protracted lower jaw position is then fixed by the pistons, this plus the substantial difficulty in eating for the first week or two, can be a heavy ordeal for a patient. It has been found to be MUCH BETTER to **avoid linking the Herbst bite jumping mechanism for one or even two weeks** whilst the patient gets used to the splints. **The patient should be started on a twice daily fluoride rinsing routine and encouraged in the highest possible standard of plaque control.**

CLINICAL MANAGEMENT

The objective is to take the mid-teenage patient from an overjet of 8-15mm into a Class III reverse overjet of 1-2mm in 6-9 months (dependent on the magnitude of the skeletal discrepancy). The reason for the over-correction is that there is always a degree of rapid rebound, 2-4mm of overjet in the first 4-6 weeks, IF the Herbst splint is removed without a thought-out retention programme.

Initially, the patient has a 3-4mm sagittal advance and 4mm of buccal opening to settle into. At the second recall visit (6-8 weeks) add a 1.5-2mm washer to the buccal pistons. These washers can be easily cut from a length of 2.0mm internal diameter tubing. The washer must be split vertically for satisfactory welding and it is important to polish this welded cuff for good tolerance. At the end of another 8-10 weeks, advance 1.5-2mm again. More than three advances have not been needed to correct any case. At the third advance a longer piston may be needed. The rate of advances will depend on the robustness of the patient and the rate of overjet change whilst avoiding unwanted labial tipping of lower incisors or uprighting of upper incisors. If lower labial procumbancy is seen, then slow down the rate of piston advances.

TECHNIQUES OF SPLINT REMOVAL

This can be a 'tender affair' for the patient and a 'slightly worrying affair' for the operator. A variety of techniques have been tried. **The lower splint is detached from the teeth some weeks before the upper.**

The operator should be well positioned and comfortably seated behind a reclined patient. The technique is to take a pair of **posterior debanding pliers** and in the premolar region on one side BEND OUT THE BUCCAL ACRYLIC. Use a precise controlled, firm but not excessive pressure and STOP IMMEDIATELY if the patient reacts briskly. Move back to the molar region on that side and repeat the firm continuous bending movement on the acrylic. Now repeat on the other side. If the splint remains firm, return to the starting side. It is advantageous to be able to remain seated behind the patient and use either hand for the appropriate side.

Suddenly the light reflectance of the splint will change as the acrylic separates from the bonding agent, usually from distally to mesially. Once this has happened bilaterally, the lower incisor capping will usually free itself. The main worry to the operator and source of discomfort to the patient is a rotational force on the lower incisors. If (very rarely) the splint will not separate, then the acrylic on the labial of $\overline{2112}$ should be weakened by bur cuts and split off first.

REMOVAL OF THE COMPOSITE

The advantage of a non-viscous light activated composite, (eg Heliosit orthodontic) is that it will split off in sheets. Again, the posterior band remover is the most useful instrument in the buccal segment area and anteriorly a watch spring scaler and Mitchell's trimmer is used. **Do not use rotary instruments.** The teeth will be slightly mobile and the gums will bleed very readily. **Remove whatever composite can be removed expeditiously** and see the patient in one week when substantial healing will have taken place and the balance of the composite should be removed. A bur may be needed for tenacious composite in some fissures.

At the lower splint removal visit, the lower splint is cleaned in an ultrasonic cleaner and **the patient CONTINUES to wear the lower splint + Herbst pistons apart from meals and a rest period each day. Very frequent tooth brushing is encouraged together with continuing the twice daily fluoride rinsing routine.**

RETENTION PHILOSOPHY

The mode of action of functional appliances in general and the Herbst appliance in particular is a matter of sharp academic debate. What is readily apparent clinically is that 15 - 16 year old patients can have serious Class II Division 1 malocclusions translated into mild Class III incisor relationships in 6-8 months. Even if significant skeletal change is taking place the extent of the occlusal change cannot be solely due to a consolidated and stable skeletal change. Additionally, although the mandible cannot be 'romanced back' from its super Class I intercuspal position to a true retruded condylor position, it is highly likely that there is an element of forward positioning of the head of the condyle on the articular eminence.

Techniques of retention are sought that allow the positive maintenance of a Class I occlusal position whilst permitting gingival health and normal caries control to be restored.

RETENTION METHODOLOGY

- First achieve a mild Class III incisor relationship with the Herbst. There is often an element of mild anterior open bite or incompleteness of overbite.

- Loosen the lower splint and remove the composite.

- **Get the patient to continue to wear the now removable lower splint PLUS the linked up pistons for part of the day (4-8 hours) and all the night.**

- Leave the lower splint out for all meals and concentrate on restoring lower gingival health.

- **As soon as the lower splint is loosened, immediately concentrate on any needed upper anterior space closure that is neccessary.** Bond any upper labial segment brackets that are required and complete upper arch space closure in 6-8 weeks.

- Whilst the upper incisors are being retracted, the mandibular dentition will drop back from a mild Class III into a Class I relationship.

- During this period the clinician should see the patient at two weekly intervals to balance the amount of wear of the lower splint and pistons with the required occlusal settling.

- When the upper spacing is as closed as is appropriate (don't fiddle about too much), remove the upper splint and any brackets, together with the composite.

- Allow three clear days for upper gingival healing.

- Then take working impressions for 'one day' upper and lower Hawley retainers to be fabricated and fitted.

- Link the retainers with either Class II elastics

   OR

- Take a maximum intercuspation wax bite and get the laboratory to link the retainers with slightly active Jasper Jumpers.

- Continue with the active sagittal retention for 6-12 months. Trim the retainers to allow vertical settling.

The above narrative concludes the description of the most commonly used style of Herbst appliance at Kingston.

HERBST EFFECT ON THE VERTICAL DIMENSION

Unlike all other Class II displacement functional appliances, **the Herbst appliance does not open the intermaxillary space.** This is probably due to the dento-alveolar intrusive effect of the acrylic overlay splints. It is possible to combine a very high pull intrusive headgear (Design Card 12A & B) with the most common upper splint design (Design Card 18) if there is an element of anterior open-bite accompanying the increased overjet. If the patient is a serious GUMMY Class II Division 1 patient and needs a Herbst, then the upper splint must have incisal tip coverage (with all its risks) plus the intrusive headgear.

THE SEMI-REMOVABLE HERBST ACRYLIC SPLINT

The upper splint is constructed and bonded as outlined above. The lower splint **starts off** being cemented to get the patient used to the system. The lower splint is made slightly deeper and cemented with a good quality fluoride containing oxyphosphate cement (eg Ormco gold). The pistons are coupled up after one week and the cemented system is worn for approximately 6 - 8 weeks. The lower splint is then loosened and the cement cleaned off the teeth. Leaving the splint out for meals, intensive brushing and fluoride rinsing rapidly restores lower gingival health and prevents the significant gingival deterioration that can take place with 6 - 8 months of a bonded splint. It does, however, imply a patient who is cooperative enough **and dextrous enough to place the pistons.** The patient then continues with the lower removable splint coupled to the upper for the further 6 months of Herbst splint therapy that is required to overcorrect the occlusion.

THE HERBST ACRYLIC SPLINT - AN OVERVIEW

Emotionally worried patients and their parents do present in the mid to late teens with serious facially handicapping malocclusions. The patients are both too late and frequently, orthodontically too jaundiced, to make a functional appliance system work for them. In spite of the level of concern, there may still be serious family reservations about having jaw surgery. The orthognathic surgery that is available may have a worrying level of morbidity and lack of a reasonably expected degree of predictability. Comparable results and treatment times may be seen for similar Class II problems treated with the Herbst appliance or a well managed orthodontic/orthognathic approach.

The Herbst acrylic splint system does have a worrying level of dental morbidity that has been outlined with complete frankness. It has been found that meticulous attention to detail will mitigate these problems to an acceptable level. This is the reason for the extensive description of technique. The Herbst appliance should not be deployed as a first choice appliance for the potentially indifferently cooperating patient in the mid or early permanent dentition. It should be thought of as a device of final orthodontic resort for the failed functional or late presenting case. With all its problems it is a superb system producing patient satisfying answers to otherwise intractable problems and needs to be included in the complete orthodontist's armamentarium.

FURTHER READING and REFERENCES - See Chapter Six

Clinical guidance on prescription

- **Prescribe for mid to late teenage, low to average FMPA, moderate to severe Class II Division 1 occlusions.**

- Consider for all Class II displacement functional appliance cases that have failed to complete, who are still **desirous** of obtaining a result, and who, **after full explanation of the potential morbidity,** ELECT to wear a Herbst splint.

- Do not restart treatment in the presence of indifferent oral health.

- Reasonable arch alignment is required prior to bonding the Herbst system.

- This may involve a preliminary phase of treatment with the visually unobtrusive ELSAA system.

- Alternatively some upper arch expansion can be achieved by gentle intraoral activation of the 'U' loop in the palatal bracing bar (Fig 18 i).

- Incisor alignment can be achieved in the later stages of the Herbst treatment by using a few anterior brackets in combination with a round 0.9mm tube inserted into the upper buccal overlay in 4|4 region (Fig 18 i & ii).

- Psychological conditioning of the patient and parent for the Herbst system requires care and TIME.

- Think through the design, particularly in relationship to the dento-alveolar adjustments required to support the sagittal arch change. These are not only tooth alignment within the arch perimeter since there may be some vertical change required also.

- Decide whether these dento-alveolar changes are required :
  1. **Prior to the Herbst** ie upper buccal segment palatal crossbites, very deep overbites or very irregular incisors.
  2. **During the Herbst** ie upper labial alignment or
  3. **After the Herbst and during retention** ie vertical settling and minor titivation of tooth positions.

- Add an intrusive headgear to a 0.051" maxillary tube for any high FMPA patients who would be appropriate for an intrusive appliance. The 0.051" tube substitutes for the 0.9mm tube (Fig 18 i) that is normally fitted. The 0.051" tube would initially be used for the headgear and laterly for any anterior space closure.

- For high FMPA patients who would be appropriate for a **buccal intrusion splint,** ie Class II Division 1 malocclusion **with very incomplete overbites and/or anterior open bites,** use the standard upper arch Herbst acrylic splint, Design 18 i.

- For high FMPA patients who would be appropriate **for the intrusive activator,** ie **gummy Class II Division 1 malocclusions with deep bites,** use a full arch Herbst acrylic splint with upper labial capping. Be very careful of upper incisor decalcification, and if a preliminary ELSAA appliance is used, add an intrusive anterior bite-plate.

- Get the patient to clean their teeth really well prior to the impressions.

- Good quality upper and lower working impressions are required **with well defined accurate gingival margins.**

- A working bite is required with 3-4mm of advance and 4mm of buccal opening.

- The techniques of a light activated bonding of the Herbst splint have been outlined at length in the section 'BONDING THE SPLINT' in the chapter text.

- Train your team, have two assistants and arrange the appointment when you are fresh and have time.

- The patient needs to be seen at four weekly intervals to check for oral health, gingival disease, splint leakage, food packing and ulceration.

- At each visit the patient should be asked to keep the teeth in contact and protrude the mandible. If 6-8mm of piston emerge forwards from the tube; **then reactivate by adding a 2mm washer.** This is likely to be every second or third visit. For the final activations add thinner washers, when longer pistons may also be needed.

- Warn the patient why they are being taken into a Class III incisal relationship with apparent mandibular prognathia.

- The 'TECHNIQUES OF SPLINT REMOVAL' and 'RETENTION METHODOLOGY' outlined in the chapter text should be followed in detail.

- Previously failed orthodontic patients who have been taken into the Herbst acrylic splint appliance, will usually have been initially delighted with the rapid reduction in retrognathia, but after six months of treatment they will want to be finished with the appliance.

- An explanation of the problems and management of potential rapid, sagittal relapse will convince most patients of the need for a further 6 months of assiduous cooperation with retention.

- **The programme of staggered debonding of first the lower,** then the upper splint, combined with upper anterior space closure, allows the opportunity for some dental adjustment of the occlusion.

- Most patients of this type will NOT consent to upper and lower full fixed appliance therapy to detail the occlusion at this stage. The clinician should plan for an acceptable treatment result with this in mind.

- Use the Hawley retainers, plus simple modification to achieve any further needed tooth movements.

Functional Component Objectives

1. Treatment of moderate to moderately severe retrognathia in the late growing face (14-17 years).
2. Maximised mandibular advance by incremental advance of the Herbst mechanism.
3. Induction of a mild Class III incisal relationship from a starting 8-15mm overjet.
4. Lateral expansion of the upper arch as appropriate.
5. Consolidation of upper arch spacing AFTER a maximised mandibular advance.
6. Post splint removal forward mandibular rotation, to compensate for within treatment induction of mild anterior openbite.
7. Retention procedures designed to minimise sagittal relapse and consolidate the orthopaedic gain.
8. Retention and treatment procedures designed to close mesio-distal incisal spacing and gain any small improvements in tooth positioning that can be obtained with the retainers.

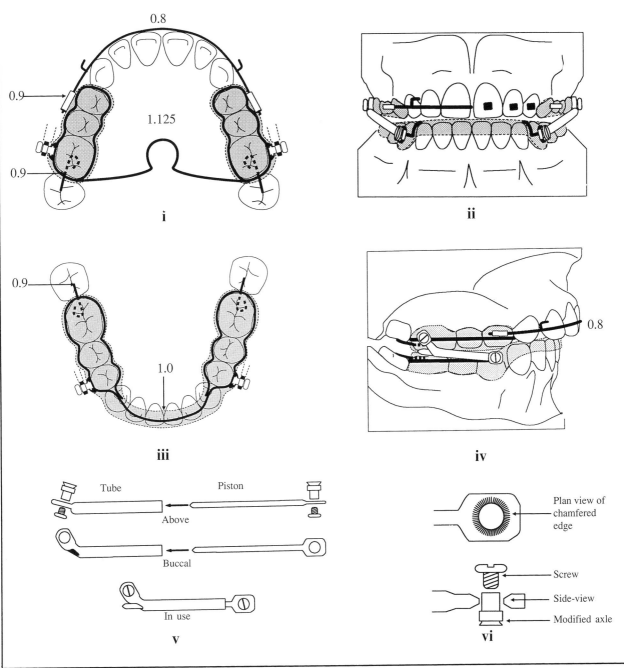

Technical guidance on construction of the UPPER splint

- On receipt of **good quality** upper and lower impressions (which should have been **recently taken**) the technician should gently rinse and gently dry the impressions.

- The first cast should be made in a good quality stone plaster to minimise distortion during fabrication.

- The impressions should be eased gently off the stone models **as soon as possible,** rinsed, blown off and immediately recast to provide duplicate working models in a mixture of 50% stone and 50% plaster.

- Articulate the first casts to the bite provided (3-4mm forward & 4mm open) on a plane line articulator, RECORD the vertical dimension.

- **The upper wire framework is bent from a single length of 1.125mm wire** on the articulated model.

- Start in the middle of the palate and bend a large omega loop. The open end of the omega should point towards the soft palate (Fig 18 i).

- The palatal bar and loop should be 5mm clear of the vault of the palate in the midline, and 2mm clear of the palatal mucosa at the gingival margins of 6|6 .. Remember that the buccal overlays will cause the teeth to sink and also the upper buccal segments may be driven distally by the Herbst mechanism. If the transpalatal bar is **too close to the mucosa of the hard palate it will impact** into the soft tissues during use.

- Also the clinician will want to be able to squeeze the base of the 'U' with a pair of Adams's pliers and the beak of the plier must be able to engage the wire a millimetre or so from the tips of the beaks.

- Use a small rectangle of wax in the mid-palate as a spacer and as a bending and positioning aid.

- The wire should pass laterally from the central omega loop to slightly mesial to the 76|67 embrasure. The wire is then curved around the distal of 6|6 and passes across the 76|67 embrasure (Fig 18 i).

- On the buccal the wire turns mesially and runs forward along the buccal of the upper buccal segment teeth.

- The wire should be **near to the occlusal surface and 1mm clear of the buccal surfaces of the teeth at the base of the buccal cusps.**

- At the mesial of 4|4 the wire turns palatally and passes through the 43|34 embrasure. The wire will rest on the embrasures.

- On the palatal the wire turns distally and travels at the same height to eventually pass to the distal of 6|6 .

- As the wire is flowing in a straightish horizontal line just below the occlusal surface, it should be gently contoured bucco-lingually in a series of flowing, sinuous but shallow curves (Fig 18 i).

- The end of the wire should be brought into contact with the palatal portion of the wire. The contact should either be a good butt joint or have 2mm of passive, but firm wire overlap and contact.

- The overlapping 2mm of wire should rest gently in contact without tension.

- At this point, check the overall form of the wire for position and shape. The wax palatal spacer is helpful and the buccal segments should be smoothly enclosed, but not quite touched by the wire. The wire will gently rest on the distal marginal ridge of 6|6 and the mesial marginal ridge of 4|4 as it travels across the embrasures. Many technicians will find this an interesting wire bending exercise!

- The wire join should be soldered.

- The axle portion of the Herbst mechanism (Fig 18 vi) is welded into position on the framework and positioned on the disto-buccal of 6|6 (Fig 18 i). A fine welding point is required to reach the bottom of the screw retaining portion. The tack welded axle is then soldered to the frame with a complete wrap around joint. Cover areas that must be clear of solder with an anti-flux.

- This soldered joint **takes a great deal of thrust and can fail.** The soldering should be of the highest quality, and a recent modification of the rim of the base of the axle (Fig 18 vi) allows solder to enter a mechanical lock on the outer rim of the axle.

- A single thickness of wax should be laid down and closely adapted to 654|456 crowns. This wax shell should be **JUST short of the gingival margins.**

- The wire framework should be warmed and then settled into the wax to its correct position.

- A doubled back 0.9mm wire is bent as an occlusal rest for 7|7 and the tag ends are waxed into position.

- 0.9mm flying EOT tubes (for the free sliding labial round 0.8 or edgewise wire) are attached to a squared off 'U' of 0.8mm wire. This is then set into the wax at a mid crown height on the buccal of 4|4 (page 91, Fig 18 i).

- **Relatively uncommonly** the clinician will want to continue an intrusive headgear system with the Herbst appliance. In this case a 0.051" tube will be required together with an intrusive whisker (see Design Card 14, technical guidance).

- Apart from the flat posterior bite planes, the buccal and palatal upper wax work is now completed.

See overleaf for technical guidance on construction of the LOWER Herbst splint.

Functional Component Objectives

1. Treatment of moderate to moderately severe retrognathia in the late growing face (14-17 years).
2. Maximised mandibular advance by incremental advance of the Herbst mechanism.
3. Induction of a mild Class III incisal relationship from a starting 8-15mm overjet.
4. Lateral expansion of the upper arch as appropriate.
5. Consolidation of upper arch spacing AFTER a maximised mandibular advance.
6. Post splint removal forward mandibular rotation, to compensate for within treatment induction of mild anterior openbite.
7. Retention procedures designed to minimise sagittal relapse and consolidate the orthopaedic gain.
8. Retention and treatment procedures designed to close mesio-distal incisal spacing and gain any small improvements in tooth positioning that can be obtained with the retainers.

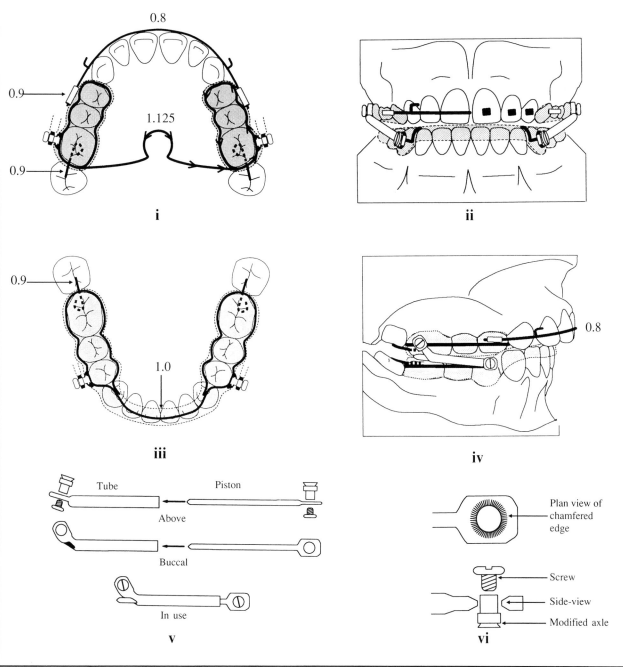

Technical guidance on construction of the LOWER splint

- **The lower wire work is made from a single length of 1.0mm wire on the articulated model.**

- The wire is gently curved on the lingual surface of $\overline{1|1}$ at one-third of the crown height below the incisal tip and then closely follows the anatomy of $\overline{321|123}$ on their lingual surfaces (Fig 18 iii).

- On the distal of $\overline{3|3}$ the wire crosses over to the buccal of the $\overline{43|34}$ embrasure and continues horizontally towards the distal, and near to the occlusal surface with a series of flowing sinuous curves in the bucco-lingual plane.

- **The wire should be near to the occlusal surface and 1mm clear of the buccal surfaces of the teeth at the base of the buccal cusps.**

- The wire enters and passes across the $\overline{76|67}$ embrasure. It then turns mesially and continues forwards with a similar contour and position to that advocated on the buccal.

- At the previously bent $\overline{43|34}$ crossover, the **lingual portion** of wire should lie passively below but in contact with the previously shaped wire on the palatal of $\overline{3|3}$ (Fig 18 iii).

- The 3mm overlap should be tack welded and soldered.

- The axle of the piston should now be tack welded and soldered onto the framework on the buccal of $\overline{4|4}$ (Fig 18 iii) in a similar manner to the upper splint.

- A sheet of wax is laid down, closely adapted to $\overline{6-1|1-6}$ to form a shell which stops **JUST short of the gingival margins** in the buccal segments and on the lingual of the lower labial segment.

- The wire frame is warmed and settled into the shell of wax.

- The tag ends of 0.9mm occlusal rests for $\overline{7|7}$ are set into the wax and the lower wax-up is completed with flat posterior bite plates (Fig 18 iii).

- The waxed Herbst frameworks are then lifted off the original models and transferred to the duplicate models for stability and to avoid distortion, during flasking and packing.

- The use of a 50% stone and 50% plaster mix (rather than using a full stone model) greatly aids deflasking.

- On the duplicate model the edges are sealed, the screws are placed in the axles, and a piece of 0.8mm wire placed in the flying EOT tubes for their stabilisation during flasking (Fig 18 i).

- The upper and lower splints are then flasked, packed and finished in a clear heat cured acrylic. **Clarity of the acrylic** is required for the light activated bonding and for seeing any loosening of the splint during use.

- After careful deflasking a high quality finish is required, with the splints tried back on the articulated master casts for any spot adjustment of the buccal bite plates. Occlusal surface grooves are cut to aid mastication.

- On the inner surface of both splints **use a small inverted cone bur to cut opposing undercuts on the inner buccal and lingual surfaces** to maximise composite to acrylic adhesion.

- On the upper splint, if the clinician requires it, fabricate a free sliding 0.8mm bow, ideal in form, 2mm from the gingival margins of $\underline{21|12}$, and with a small upward crank for levelling some 6-8mm mesial to the $\underline{4|4}$ tubes. Solder a small hook for elastic traction at the crank.

- Screw on the tubes, bring the splints into occlusion and mark the tube lengths 1.5mm distal to the $\overline{4|4}$ axle, shorten, smooth and polish.

- Place the pistons, engage the tubes and **shorten the projecting end of the pistons** so that they are in line with the centre of the upper upper axles, **round and polish well.** If the pistons are left too long, this is a potent cause of ulceration.

- Since the tubes and pistons are frequently slightly asymmetric it is **very important to be able to distinguish between the right and left tube and piston.** It is suggested that the right assembly is colour coded with red nail varnish.

Functional Component Objectives

1. Treatment of moderate to moderately severe retrognathia in the late growing face (14-17 years).
2. Maximised mandibular advance by incremental advance of the Herbst mechanism.
3. Induction of a mild Class III incisal relationship from a starting 8-15mm overjet.
4. Lateral expansion of the upper arch as appropriate.
5. Consolidation of upper arch spacing AFTER a maximised mandibular advance.
6. Post splint removal forward mandibular rotation, to compensate for within treatment induction of mild anterior openbite.
7. Retention procedures designed to minimise sagittal relapse and consolidate the orthopaedic gain.
8. Retention and treatment procedures designed to close mesio-distal incisal spacing and gain any small improvements in tooth positioning that can be obtained with the retainers.

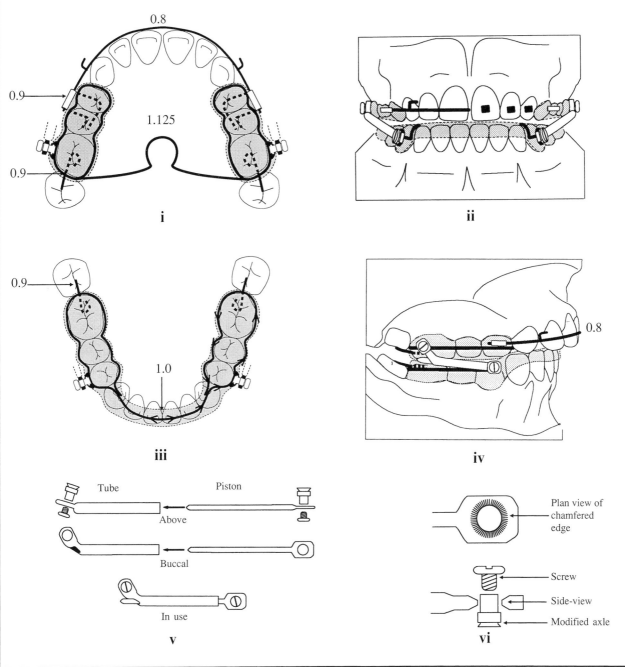

i

ii

iii

iv

Tube · Piston
Above
Buccal
In use

v

Plan view of chamfered edge
Screw
Side-view
Modified axle

vi

CHAPTER SIX

FURTHER READING AND SOME 'KEY' REFERENCES

The reader will have noticed that there are very few references to the literature throughout the text, and that at the end of the introduction to each chapter there has been a reference to this particular chapter. There have been a variety of reasons for this :

- Where important clinical techniques have been originated by other authors eg Andresen, Clark, Fränkel, Herbst, Mew etc, this has been acknowledged within the text.

- Some of the techniques have, however, evolved within the Kingston Hospital Orthodontic Department.

- Both 'homegrown' and 'imported' functional appliance techniques have been refined, moulded and sometimes blended, as a consequence of their testing on many serious malocclusions by a variety of trainees, of varying aptitude.

- The distillation of a decade and a half of experience is now presented as a successful treatment system, that will allow an average but well motivated clinician to treat all serious Class II malocclusions in the growing face of the cooperative patient.

- **This fact is the principle reference basis on which this atlas rests.**

- Where Kingston data and techniques have been published, or are in press, then these references are noted in the reading list.

- Some data has been presented as 'read papers' to the British Society for the Study of Orthodontics, but have not been written up (the author apologises).

- The author wished to leave the text relatively uncluttered, so that it could be assessed for itself.

- Suggestions for further reading with some references appropriate to each chapter are printed overleaf.

- The list of references is not intended to be exhaustive, rather it is designed to give a serious student an introductory overview to each of the chapter topics.

- The author would apologise to other authors who might rightly feel that their own particular article(s) had been unwisely excluded from the condensed list.

- The first section of the references is chosen to give an overview of the philosophy behind the decision to use 'functional appliances' within the armamentarium of the "Compleat Orthodontist" (with apologies to Izaak W).

- Literature references as to the value of functional appliance systems, may be broadly divided into those in favour and those against.

- The negative references have been largely excluded since they simply do not fit in with the 'Overview' that the author has gained in the successful use of these systems on many, many patients.

- The "Compleat Orthodontist" seeking to successfully and continually 'land' serious malocclusion will require, **enthusiasm, knowledge,** the skills borne of **experience and constant practice,** together with **determined perseverence.**

FUNCTIONAL APPLIANCE PHILOSOPHY - Contributions to an 'Overview'

1. **Adams, CP.** *The design and construction of removable orthodontic appliances, 4th Edition.* Bristol, John Wright & Sons, 1979.

2. **Carels, C and van der Linden, FPGM.** Concepts on functional appliances' mode of action. *Am. J. Orthod.* 92: 162-168, 1987.

3. **Isaacson, KG, Reed, RT and Stephens, CD.** *Functional Orthodontic Appliances.* Oxford, Blackwell Scientific Publications, 1990.

4. **McNamara, JA, Connelly, TG and McBride, MC.** Histological studies of temperomandibular joint adaptations. In : *Determinants of mandibular form and growth,* Monograph No 4, Craniofacial growth series. 209-227. McNamara, JA. Centre for human growth and development, University of Michigan, Ann Arbor, Michigan, 1975.

5. **McNamara, JA and Carlson, D.** Quantitative analysis of temperomandibular joint adaptations to protrusive function. *Am. J. Orthod.* 76: 593-611, 1979.

6. **McNamara, JA.** Functional determinents of craniofacial size and shape. *Eur. J. Orthod.* 2: 131-159, 1980.

7. **McNamara, JA, Hinton, RJ and Hoffman, DL.** Adaptation to protrusive function in young adult monkeys. *Am. J. Orthod.* 82: 288-298, 1982.

8. **McNamara, JA and Bryan, FA.** Long-term adaptations to protrusive function : An experimental study on Macaca Mulatta. *Am. J. Orthod.* 92: 98-108, 1987.

9. **Orton, HS and Jones, SP.** Lower second and third molars - their correction when mesially impacted. *Oral Health.* 77: No 9: 29-32, 1987.

10. **Petrovic, A, Stutzman, J and Oudet, C.** Control processes in the post-natal growth of the mandibular condylar cartilage. In: *Determinents of mandibular form and growth,* Monograph No 4, Craniofacial growth series, McNamara, J A. University of Michigan, Ann Arbor, Michigan, 1975.

11. **Petrovic, A, Stutzman, J and Gasson, N.** The final length of the mandible : is it genetically predetermined? In: *Craniofacialbiology,* Monograph No 10, Craniofacial growth series, Carlson, D S, University of Michigan, Ann Arbor, Michigan, 1981.

12. **Stöckli, PW and Willert, HG.** Tissue reaction in the temporomandibular joint resulting from anterior displacement of the mandible in the monkey. *Am. J. Orthod.* 60: 142- 155, 1971.

13. **Stöckli, PW and Dietrich, VC.** Experimental and clinical findings following functional forward displacement of the mandible. *Trans of the E.O.S.,* 435-442, 1973.

14. **Teuscher, U.** A growth related concept for Skeletal Class II treatment. *Am. J. Orthod.* 74: 258-275, 1978.

15. **Woodside, DG, Metaxas, A and Altuna, G.** The influence of functional appliance therapy on glenoid fossa remodeling. *Am. J. Orthod.* 92: 181-198, 1987.

FRANKEL APPLIANCES - Chapter 1

1. **Eirew, HL, McDowell, F and Phillips, JG.** The functional regulator of Frankel. *B. J. Orthod.* 3: 67-74, 1976.

2. **Eirew, HL., McDowell, F andPhillips, JG.** The Frankel appliance : Avoidance of lower incisor proclination. *B. J. Orthod.* 8: 189-192, 1981.

3. **Fränkel, R.** The treatment of Class II Division 1 malocclusion with functional correctors. *Am. J. Orthod.* 55: 265-275, 1969.

4. **Fränkel, R.** Maxillary retrusion in Class III cases and treatment with the functional corrector III. *Trans of the E.O.S.,* 249-259, 1970.

5. **Fränkel, R.** A functional approach to orofacial orthopaedics. *B. J. Orthod.* 7: 41-51, 1980.

6. **Fränkel, R. and Fränkel, Ch.** *Orofacial orthopedics with the function regulator.* Basle, Karger, 1989.

7. **Loh, MK and Kerr, WJS.** The function regulator III : Effects and indications for use. *B. J. Orthod.* 12: 153-157, 1985.

8. **McNamara, JA, Bookstein, FL and Shaughnessy, TG.** Skeletal and dental changes following functional regulator therapy on Class II patients. *Am. J. Orthod.* 88: 91-110, 1985.

9. **McWade, RA, Mamandras, AH and Stuart-Hunter, W.** The effects of Frankel II treatment on arch width and arch perimeter. *Am. J. Orthod.* 92: 313-320, 1987.

10. **Owen, AH.** Morphological changes in the sagittal dimension using the Frankel appliance. *Am. J. Orthod.* 80: 573-603, 1981.

11. **Robertson, NRE.** An examination of treatment changes in children treated with the functional regulator of Frankel. *Am. J. Orthod.* 83: 299-310, 1983.

ELSAA's - Chapter 2

1. **Adams, CP.** *The design and construction of removable orthodontic appliances, 4th Edition.* Bristol, John Wright & Sons, 48-62, 1979.

2. **Haas, AJ.** Palatal expansion : Just the beginning of dentofacial orthopedics. *Am. J. Orthod.* 57: 219-255, 1977.

3. **Hicks, E.** Slow maxillary expansion : a clinical study of the skeletal verses the dental response to low magnitude force. *Am. J. Orthod.* 73: 121-141, 1978.

4. **Mew, JRC.** Semi-rapid maxillary expansion. *B. Dent. J.* 143: 301-306, 1977.

5. **Orton, HS and Carter, NE.** Initial management of first molar extraction cases. *J. Clin. Orthod.* 12: No 4: 230-234, 1988.

ACTIVATORS - Chapter 3

1. **Ahlgren, J and Laurin, C.** Late results of activator treatment : a cephalometric study. *B. J. Orthod.* 3: 181-187, 1976.

2. **Eirew, H.** The bionator. *B. J. Orthod.* 8: 33-36, 1981.

3. **Forsberg, CM and Odenrick, L.** Skeletal and soft tissue response to activator treatment. *Eur. J. Orthod.* 3: 247-253, 1981.

4. **Harvold, E and Vargervik, K.** Morphogenetic response to activator treatment. *Am. J. Orthod.* 60: 478-490, 1971.

5. **Harvold, E.** The activator in interceptive orthodontics. *St Louis,* Mosby. 92-94, 1974.

6. **Leuder, HU.** Effects of activator treatment : evidence for two different types of reaction. *Eur. J. Orthod.* 3: 205-222, 1981.

7. **Mörndal, O.** The effect on the incisor teeth of activator treatment : a follow-up study. *B. J. Orthod.* 11: 214-220, 1984.

8. **Orton, HS and McDonald FM.** A simple sectional canine retraction technique using the properties of nickel-titanium rectangular wire. *Eur. J. Orthod.* 7: 120-126, 1985.

9. **Pancherz, H.** A cephalometric analysis of skeletal and dental changes contributing to Class II correction in activator treatment. *Am. J. Orthod.* 85: 125-134, 1984.

10. **Reed, RT and Hathorn, IS.** The activator. *B. J. Orthod.* 55: 75-80, 1978.

11. **Weislander, L and Lagerström, L.** The effects of activator treatment on Class II malocclusions. *Am. J. Orthod.* 75: 20-26, 1979.

12. **Woodside, D.** The activator. In : Saltzman, JA : *Orthodontics in daily practice.* Philadelphia, 1974, Lippincott, JB.

'INTRUSIVE' FUNCTIONAL APPLIANCES - Chapter 4

1. **Bass, NM.** Dentofacial orthopaedics in the correction of Class II malocclusion. *B. J. Orthod.* 9: 3-31, 1982.

2. **Blechman, AM.** Magnetic force systems in orthodontics. *Am. J. Orthod.* 87: 201-210, 1985.

3. **Caldwell, SF, Hymas, TA and Timm, TA.** Maxillary traction splint : A cephalometric evaluation. *Am. J. Orthod.* 85: 376-384, 1984.

4. **Chaconas, FJ, Caputo, AA and Davis, JC.** The effect of orthopedic forces on the cranio-facial complex, utilising cervical and headgear forces. *Am. J. Orthod.* 69: 527-539, 1976.

5. **Clark, WJ.** The twin block traction technique. *E. J. Orthod.* 4: 129-138, 1982.

6. **Dellinger, EL.** A clinical assessment of the active vertical corrector - A non-surgical alternative for skeletal open bite treatment. *Am. J. Orthod.* 89: 428-436, 1986.

7. **Droschl, H and Tuenge, RH.** The effect of heavy orthopedic forces on the maxilla in the growing Saimiri scieureus (squirrel monkey). *Am. J. Orthod.* 63: 449-461, 1973.

8. **Elder, JR and Tuenge, RJ.** Cephalometric and histological changes produced by extra-oral high pull traction to the maxilla of Macaca mulatta. *Am. J. Orthod.* 66: 599-617, 1974

'INTRUSIVE' FUNCTIONAL APPLIANCES - Chapter 4 (Contd)

9. **Elder, JR and Tuenge, RJ.** Post treatment changes following extra-oral high pull traction to the maxilla of Macaca mulatta. *Am. J. Orthod.* 66: 618-643, 1974.

10. **Fotis, V, Melsen, B and Williams, S.** Vertical control as an important ingredient in the treatment of severe sagittal discrepancies. *Am. J. Orthod.* 86: 224-232, 1984.

11. **Henry, HL.** An experimental study of external force application to the maxillary complex. In : *Factors affecting the growth of the midface*, Monograph No 6, Craniofacial growth series, 301-325. McNamara, JA.Centre for human growth and development, University of Michigan, Ann Arbor, Michigan, 1976.

12. **Levin, RI.** Activator headgear therapy. *Am. J. Orthod.* 87: 91-109, 1985.

13. **Orton, HS, Slattery, DA and Orton, S.** The treatment of severe gummy Class II Division 1 malocclusion using the maxillary intrusion splint. Submitted for publication in *Am. J. Orthod* 1989.

14. **Thurow, RC.** Craniofacial orthopedic corrections with en-masse dental control. *Am. J. Orthod.* 68: 601-624, 1975.

15. **Van Beek, H.** Overjet correction by a combined headgear and activator. *Eur. J. Orthod.* 4: 279-290, 1982.

THE HERBST APPLIANCE - Chapter 5

1. **Herbst, E.** *Atlas und Grundriss der Zannartlichen Orthopädie.* Munich, Lehmann, J. F. 1910.

2. **Howe, RP.** The Herbst appliance : an alternative design using a bonded splint. *J. Clin. Orthod.* 16: 663-667, 1982.

3. **Howe, RP.** Updating the bonded Herbst appliance. *J. Clin. Orthod.* 17: 122-124, 1983.

4. **Howe, RP.** The acrylic splint Herbst : problem solving. *J. Clin. Orthod.* 18: 497-501, 1984.

5. **Langford, NM Jr,** The Herbst appliance. *J. Clin. Orthod.* 15: 58-61, 1982.

6. **Langford, NM Jr,** Updating fabrication of the Herbst appliance. *J. Clin. Orthod.* 16: 173-174, 1982.

7. **McNamara, JA and Howe, RP.** Clinical management of the acrylic splint. *Am. J. Orthod.* 94: 142-149, 1988.

8. **Pancherz, H.** The effect of continuous bite-jumping on the dentofacial complex : A follow-up study after Herbst appliance treatment of Class II malocclusions. *Eur. J. Orthod.* 3: 49-60, 1981.

9. **Pancherz, H.** The mechanism of Class II correction in Herbst appliance treatment. *Am. J. Orthod.* 82: 105-114, 1982.

10. **Pancherz, H.** The Herbst appliance - Its biological effects and clinical use. *Am. J. Orthod.* 87: 1-20, 1985.

11. **Pancherz, H.** Mandibular anchorage in Herbst treatment. *Eur. J. Orthod.* 10: 149-164, 1988.

WIRE DIAMETER & GAUGE CONVERSION CHART

For stainless steel wires used in fabricating orthodontic functional appliances.

- There are internationally many different measures, or gauges, used for the measurement of wire diameter.
- The metric system is used for most of Europe.
- The metric system (millimetres) has superseded the Imperial system (inches) in the United Kingdom for dental laboratory products.
- The whole of the large North American market uses the Brown & Sharpe or 'AMERICAN GAUGE' for orthodontic wire technology.
- The Imperial system (inches) predominates in the USA fixed appliance market and this has dominated the European and Pacific countries fixed appliance market.
- In Europe it leads to the anomaly of a curious mixture of metric and Imperial measurement in orthodontic jargon.
- The diagrams are thus primarily labelled in millimetres, but there is the **American gauge equivalent of each size that is mentioned at the bottom of each page.**
- To facilitate a more comprehensive comparison for all of the wire sizes mentioned, the appended table allows a ready conversion **from millimetres to American gauge,** but will also allow a conversion to Imperial (inches) or to Standard Wire Gauge.
- It should be remembered however that it is not only **the diameter** but also **the type** of wire used that will affect its qualities.
- The most important qualities are the STIFFNESS (modulus) and the BRITTLENESS (fragility) of the wire type selected to fabricate the orthodontic appliance.
- The wire used at Kingston is an 18:8, chrome:cobalt stainless steel. It is a **medium drawn wire*** rather than an extra hard drawn wire.
- In orthodontic wire technology it is better generally to avoid the extra-hard drawn (and frequently brittle) wires.
- As a general rule in orthodontic wire technology, if added resilience is needed, increase the wire **diameter** rather than the modulus of the wire.

Stainless Steel Wire Diameter/Gauges and Conversion Chart**

Metric	American Gauge	Imperial	Standard Wire Gauge
0.7	21	0.0276	22
0.8	20	0.0320	21
0.9	19	0.0354	20
1.0	18	0.0394	19
1.125	17	0.0443	18/19
1.25	16	0.0492	18
1.5	15	0.0590	16/17
1.8	13	0.0720	15

*   Wire fabricated by K C Smith & Co, Port Talbot, Wales. United Kingdom.
** Source : Camm, FJ. *Practical Mechanics Handbook*. London, Newnes, G. 8th Ed 1966.

Index